Becoming an Expert Caregiver

Carework in a Changing World

Amy Armenia, Mignon Duffy, and
Kim Price-Glynn, Series Editors

The rise of scholarly attention to care has accompanied greater public concern about aging, health care, child care, and labor in a global world. Research on care is happening across disciplines—in sociology, economics, political science, philosophy, public health, social work, and others—with numerous research networks and conferences developing to showcase this work. Care scholarship brings into focus some of the most pressing social problems facing families today. To study care is also to study the future of work, as issues of carework are intertwined with the forces of globalization, technological development, and the changing dynamics of the labor force. Care scholarship is also at the cutting edge of intersectional analyses of inequality, as carework is often at the very core of understanding gender, race, migration, age, disability, class, and international inequalities.

Sophie Bourgault, Maggie FitzGerald, and Fiona Robinson, eds., Decentering Epistemologies and Challenging Privilege: Critical Care Ethics Perspectives
Cara A. Chiaraluce, Becoming an Expert Caregiver: How Structural Flaws Shape Autism Carework and Community
Mignon Duffy, Amy Armenia, and Kim Price-Glynn, eds., From Crisis to Catastrophe: Care, COVID, and Pathways to Change
Fumilayo Showers, Migrants Who Care: West Africans Working and Building Lives in U.S. Health Care

Becoming an Expert Caregiver

~

How Structural Flaws Shape Autism Carework and Community

CARA A. CHIARALUCE

Rutgers University Press
New Brunswick, Camden, and Newark, New Jersey
London and Oxford

Rutgers University Press is a department of Rutgers, The State University of New Jersey, one of the leading public research universities in the nation. By publishing worldwide, it furthers the University's mission of dedication to excellence in teaching, scholarship, research, and clinical care.

Library of Congress Cataloging-in-Publication Data
Names: Chiaraluce, Cara A., author.
Title: Becoming an expert caregiver : how structural flaws shape autism carework & community / Cara A. Chiaraluce.
Description: New Brunswick, New Jersey : Rutgers University Press, [2025] | Series: Carework in a changing world | Includes bibliographical references and index.
Identifiers: LCCN 2024016313 | ISBN 9781978831902 (paperback) | ISBN 9781978831919 (hardcover) | ISBN 9781978831926 (epub) | ISBN 9781978831940 (pdf)
Subjects: LCSH: Parents of autistic children. | Autistic children. | Autistic children—Care. | Autism.
Classification: LCC HQ773.8 .C45 2025 | DDC 649/.1526—dc23/eng/20240719
LC record available at https://lccn.loc.gov/2024016313

A British Cataloging-in-Publication record for this book is available from the British Library.

Copyright © 2025 by Cara A. Chiaraluce
All rights reserved
No part of this book may be reproduced or utilized in any form or by any means, electronic or mechanical, or by any information storage and retrieval system, without written permission from the publisher. Please contact Rutgers University Press, 106 Somerset Street, New Brunswick, NJ 08901. The only exception to this prohibition is "fair use" as defined by U.S. copyright law.

References to internet websites (URLs) were accurate at the time of writing. Neither the author nor Rutgers University Press is responsible for URLs that may have expired or changed since the manuscript was prepared.

♾ The paper used in this publication meets the requirements of the American National Standard for Information Sciences—Permanence of Paper for Printed Library Materials, ANSI Z39.48-1992.
rutgersuniversitypress.org

For Sam and Sofia

Contents

	Introduction	1
1.	Autism Complexities: Competing Paradigms and Historical Context	23
2.	Tracing Transformation: The Birth of the Expert Caregiver	41
3.	Making Sense of Difference: Building the Expert Caregiver Toolkit	67
4.	Transcending the Private Sphere: Extending Carework into the Community	95
5.	Potentials and Limits of Expert Caregiving: Community Carework and Medicalization	108
6.	"I Need Some Air Down Here and Nobody Is Noticing": Caring about the Expert Caregiver	125
	Appendix A: Methodology and Caregiver Demographics	137
	Appendix B: Interview Schedule	145
	Acknowledgments	147
	References	149
	Index	161

Becoming an Expert Caregiver

Introduction

"The hardest thing is dealing with the rest of the world. And we kind of accommodate our lives around that. But the rest of the world doesn't." These poignant words were spoken to me by Charlotte, a mother and primary caregiver of a five-year-old autistic boy, in my very first interview with autism caregivers. Her words reference the structural arrangements of our world that shape autism carework today. In the chapters that follow, you will hear from fifty primary caregivers of autistic and neurodivergent children who illuminate the process through which lay women become expert caregivers to provide the best care for their children. Expert caregiving captures an intensification of traditional family carework—meeting dependents' financial, emotional, and physical needs—that transcends the walls of one's private home and family, and challenges the strict boundaries between many worlds: lay and professional, family and work, private and public, medical and social, and individual and society. The process of becoming an expert caregiver spotlights several interesting paradoxes in sociological literature, particularly regarding gender, family, and medicalization, and often-forgotten structural flaws in "the rest of the world."

The expert caregiver emerges from an insufficient and fragmented social safety net that places the overwhelming burden of care on the shoulders of individual caregivers and their families. Specifically, the expert caregiver is shaped by cumulative frustrations in U.S. care systems, particularly in education and health care, and constraining flaws in entrenched cultural ideals of gender, family, and ability. What is more, these structural flaws and cultural assumptions are largely invisible to the dominant neurotypical eye.

The latest statistics from the Centers for Disease Control and Prevention (Centers for Disease Control and Prevention [CDC], 2023) hold that one in thirty-six American children is diagnosed with autism, which is more than a tenfold increase in prevalence in the last forty years.[1] Additionally, the CDC and the Health Resources and Services Administration (HRSA) estimate that one in six, or about 17 percent, of U.S. children aged three through seventeen years has one or more developmental disabilities like autism. It is evident that the population of children with developmental disabilities, and the families who care for them, is growing in the United States. Despite the increasing population and attention to autism, it continues to be rife with uncertainty and controversy.

At the time of writing, there are two competing paradigms that guide fundamentally different orientations to autism: the biomedical model and the social model of disability. The biomedical model defines autism as a bioneurological developmental disorder that varies in severity, characterized by persistent deficits in social communication and repetitive patterns of behavior, interests, or activities (American Psychiatric Association [APA], 2013). In contrast to the idea of autism as a medical disorder that can be diagnosed, treated, and potentially cured, the social model of disability defines autism as a neurotype that functions as a category of disability and identity; it refers to a different form of brain wiring, not a disordered or flawed one.

Therefore, tensions and ambiguity (both professional and lay) exist in the fundamental orientations to autism that significantly affect the caring experience and provide the backdrop for

---

1. Previously, in 2018, the Autism and Developmental Disabilities Monitoring (ADDM) Network, a program funded by CDC, estimated that one in forty-four children are autistic. See Maenner et al., 2020.

understanding caregivers' experiences in this book, which are detailed further in chapter 1. While living within these larger societal tensions, families are seeking information, support, and social inclusion to maximize the quality of life and well-being for their children and themselves.

Within this contested landscape, an expert caregiver manages a household and strives to meet the expectations of a good mother while also taking on vast informally trained professional roles that expand carework outside the private domestic sphere of home and family. She is a lay diagnostician; teacher; social worker; speech, physical, and occupational therapist; skilled nurse; advocate; change maker; community builder; partner; and mother who frequently works outside the home in the paid labor market, all while completing the lion's share of traditional domestic duties.

How do individual caregivers do all of this, why, and what are some of their impacts at individual and community levels? I wanted to learn more about the different paths that women take to becoming expert caregivers, how they navigate complex formal systems saturated with frustratingly long waitlists and gatekeepers that delay action and aid (i.e., waitlists for specialists, diagnostic evaluations, and support services), what motivations and goals drive their behaviors to take on an array of professional roles and extend their caring labor outside the home, and the benefits and burdens involved in each step of their caring journeys for themselves, their children and families, and their communities.

I use a narrative approach to deeply understand the autism caring experience from each caregiver's perspective. I investigate how lay caregivers construct and characterize the complex autism caring experience, and the cultural discourses and narrative tools they draw on to make sense of their experiences and express their personal stories within their homes and local communities. Each chapter casts a sociological eye on autism-specific carework as unpaid labor that is both self-interested and prosocial, deeply personal and a public project entrenched in power dynamics.

More specifically, the chapters that follow unpack the *what* (actual practices, roles, and forms of caring labor that constitute expert caregiving), the *how* (through what means and avenues they become expert caregivers), the *why* (individual rationales and structural roots that guide movements on the path to becoming expert caregivers), and the *so what* (consequences associated with expert caregiving at both the individual and community levels). Flowing in a scalar fashion from micro to macro, together these chapters make typically invisible and assumed aspects of dominant neurotypical social and institutional life visible. Analysis highlights systematic flaws in the fragmented, privatized, and therefore frustrating systems of care that lead to the intensification of carework and drive the creation of the expert caregiver whose labor extends far beyond the home and family. Further, expert caregiving emerges as a compelling space to transcend seemingly fixed boundaries between several worlds: lay and professional, private and public, individual (self) and society, family and work, feminine and masculine, and unpaid labor and paid work.

First, the process of becoming an expert caregiver begins on the micro level, where social experiences of exclusion and ableism deeply impact individual caregivers' personal sense of self-identity. Ableism is defined as "a set of beliefs or practices that devalue and discriminate against people with physical, intellectual, or psychiatric disabilities and often rests on the assumption that disabled people need to be 'fixed' in one form or the other" (Smith, n.d.). The "fixing" associated with brain-based disabilities, like autism, involves the foundational assumption that all brains are wired in one way, and this one way is deemed correct and "normal."

Then, caregivers try to make sense of their child's atypical traits and missed or delayed developmental milestones and decide what to do—if anything at all. Since the medical model is the predominant cultural paradigm for understanding autism, the caregivers in this study first turn to their pediatricians for help. "Something in their gut" or their "maternal instincts" tell them their child is "different," so they soldier on within the medical model to understand their child's behaviors and set off on a diagnostic journey.

After navigating winding obstacles to receive a medical diagnosis, most caregivers describe feeling very alone and "in the dark." The doctor says, "Your child is autistic," "We'll check back in six months to see how things are going," and "Here is a list of numbers to call for information and to set up therapies." This diagnostic moment is deeply unsatisfying for the caregivers who have been searching for answers or information or validation for years. The average length from identification of puzzling traits or red-flag behaviors to diagnosis was two years in this sample.

In the United States, autism can be diagnosed as early as two years by several different medical professionals, notably developmental or behavioral pediatricians, neurologists, and child psychiatrists. Research shows that initial concerns are typically expressed or identified at children's eighteen- and twenty-four-month well-child visits with pediatricians. However, the mean age of diagnosis is 3.5 to 5 years. Therefore, the journey to the autism diagnosis, also referred to as a "diagnostic odyssey," takes anywhere from roughly two to three and half years, nationally. There are multiple reasons to explain this time gap, many of which are explored in this book, though in the United States they boil down to "a backlog of patients waiting to be seen and a lack of qualified providers" (Gordon-Lipkin, Foster, & Peacock, 2016). This delayed and unstandardized diagnostic process adds to the caring labor experienced by caregivers, which you'll hear about in the chapters that follow. Although the number of autistic children is steadily rising, and autism is an increasingly recognized developmental disability, streamlined and easily accessible knowledge and resources are still difficult to attain.

Frustrated by ineffective interactions with institutions, families are forced to turn away from professionals, and instead embark on the journey to become experts themselves. Caregivers are frustrated with the lack of support and mixed messages from professionals, frustrated with the "wait-and-see" approach, and frustrated with friends and family "not getting it," dismissing their concerns, and excluding them from normative family spaces and events. These accumulating frustrations drive the search for resources, skill-building, and social inclusion that are at the heart of the contemporary expert caregiver and the caregiver's engagement in community carework.

To address these frustrations and overcome obstacles in the caring experience, caregivers learn entirely new skill sets, bodies of knowledge, and ways of interacting and communicating, which become part of the expert caregiver toolkit. Throughout this process, you'll see when private in-home carework duties transgress typically strict public/private, paid/unpaid, and lay/expert boundaries, causing caregivers to assume a variety of formal professional roles, albeit unpaid, unacknowledged, and often alone. Further, once caregivers feel informed and capable of meeting their child's needs, the process of becoming an expert caregiver starts to transcend the boundaries of the private home and family to include engagement in the local community and broader institutional realm.

Accordingly, a hallmark of expert caregiving is the extension of caring labor outside the home and into the surrounding community, largely through prosocial advocacy practices aimed at building inclusive communities and increasing access to social capital for all families with neurodivergent children. I refer to "community carework" as a prosocial extension of intensive caring labor outside the private sphere and into organizational and institutional arenas. Community carework makes visible the additional unpaid work caregivers are doing at the organizational and institutional levels, largely outside the home and in a variety of public settings, such as organizing educational resource fairs and fundraising events, grant writing for local nonprofit groups, advocating for school trainings, extensive group administration (i.e., maintaining email listservs and digital resource tools), mentoring other caregivers, volunteering at autism awareness events, and for some, direct action to call for policy change. In doing so, we see what caring at the community level looks like and how the expert caregiver toolkit continues to expand and professionalize, challenging hierarchical bounds between lay/expert and private/public realms.

Importantly, these broader community-oriented administrative, educational, and social change practices are not typically considered part of paid or unpaid carework activities. Therefore, community carework expands traditional definitions of carework and emphasizes the ways individual everyday family labor can operate as a significant public project that is integrated within local communities and institutions.

For many, the necessity of becoming an expert caregiver is rooted in cumulative experiences of social exclusion and family marginalization in everyday life and institutional arenas, which result from flawed care systems and dominant constructions of disability as "deviant" or "bad." In this vein, this book also builds on literature in disability studies and motherhood and medicalization by showing how, in the attempt to navigate ableist structures, secure services, challenge dominant lay/expert knowledge production, and cultivate more inclusive social experiences, caregivers can simultaneously enable and challenge medicalization.

The paradox here is striking; caregivers pose as both agents of and obstacles to medicalization. Parents absolutely need formal medical recognition and diagnosis to receive life-altering services and rights for their children, but in doing so, they actively expand the jurisdiction of medicine into their private homes, schools, and everyday life. Sophisticated expert caregivers learn how to access and use medicalization to their children's benefit, while also knowing when, where, and how to push back against medical dominance. Unpacking the paradoxical and complicated relationship between medicalization and expert caregiving is an important aspect of this study and highlights the limitations associated with expert caregiving.

Lastly, I still think about the women in this study. Years later, I can vividly remember sitting at the kitchen table, watching a young mom put on the kettle for tea with one hand while holding a baby on her hip with the other. Her son was in the background bouncing on a trampoline with a tutor as she, in painstaking detail, walked through a typical day and shared with me what autism meant for her and her family. These conversations, and the extreme vulnerability and honesty with which each woman spoke, have stayed with me.

In full transparency, I completed all the research for this book before I became a mother myself; I've been a sociologist for far longer than I've been a mother. Now, I'm a mother of two children under six, one born in the pandemic, whose birth coincides with the production of this book. My personal and professional worlds have collided in recent years and have been synthesized in writing this book. When my son was not talking at one and a half years old and no one else was concerned, I thought about these women. When I first noticed signs of stimming and other atypical developmental delays in my son, I thought about these women. When I brought my concerns to the pediatrician and asked to see a developmental specialist, he referred me to a social worker for parenting help instead. I thought about these women. And, after waiting months for a comprehensive neuropsychological evaluation, the results were inconclusive, and therefore, we wait and see. I continue to think about these women and their children to this day.

The knowledge I gained from the caregivers in this study has afforded me structure and validation in my own family's journey with developmental delays and puzzling traits in early childhood. For this, I am personally indebted to the women in this study, and they and their families deserve to be heard.

The Expert Caregiver and Positionality

The overwhelming majority of families in this study self-identify as monoracial white, heterosexual, married, and middle class—families that possess a variety of social privileges and match closely with the traditional nuclear family norm or Standard North American Family (SNAF). According to Dorothy Smith (1993), the Standard North American Family is an ideological code defined in terms of both family structure—a heterosexual, legally married couple with healthy, able-bodied children—and in terms of family roles, a gendered division of labor within the family and home in which women oversee the domestic labor, including all child and home care, and men work outside the home as primary breadwinners.

As an ideological code, this one conceptualization of the family operates as a universal norm through which all ideas of family, motherhood, and child-rearing are understood and constructed. In other words, the traditional nuclear family ideal is the reference point and center through which both individuals and institutions conceptualize and understand typical family roles and structure. Throughout this book, you'll hear how this highly romanticized idea of family becomes the ideal through which mothers start interrogating ideas of normality and deviance.

Caring for autistic children forces caregivers to confront their own positionality—who they are and their location in society. They do so through normative discourses and *ideals* (not necessarily *real* ideas) of family. Using narrative reflection, caregivers commonly find that they no longer fit neatly within their previously embodied social categories of caregiver, mother, wife, sister, or professional and that the dominant heteronormative white, middle-class frameworks through which they always made sense of themselves, their lives, and their imagined futures no longer match their realities. In other words, as a result of experiencing bias based on their children's disability status, they are able to see and acknowledge their privileges in ways that they never did before. The disability status of their children becomes a lens through which caregivers experience social marginalization and public disapproval, while they may maintain race and class privileges.

This process of disenfranchisement from discourses and narratives of family are often discussed in the literature on single mothers and LGBTQ+ families. However, the link to families with disabilities and chronic disorders is undertheorized. Therefore, this book attempts to address this gap by showing how caring for neurodivergent children is a nuanced deviation from heteronormative ideas of family, which can lead to significant feelings of social exclusion and marginalization for mothers, who possess other forms of social advantage. As you will see in chapter 2, caregivers then turn to symbolic resources and community-building interventions to chip away at the dominance of the ideal American family and write new, more inclusive and realistic codes for understanding contemporary American family life.

Further, the majority of women in this study self-identify as cisgender, white, middle-class, heterosexual, married, native English speakers. Seventy-two percent are college educated and fifty-six percent of participants work outside of the home in either full- or part-time paid jobs. These demographics clearly do not represent the diversity of families with autistic children, which means that the narratives shared in this book largely represent a specific point of view. The participants in this study were recruited via a variety of advertisements posted at local public libraries, parks, health clinics, and autism community and advocacy groups. After speaking with each volunteer, I employed a snowball sampling method, which allows for peer referrals to help gain access to more people and is useful for hard-to-reach populations.

Central to a snowballing technique is that friends recommend friends. We live highly segregated lives—we often work, play, learn, and live next door to people who look like us. Therefore, one way to explain the homogeneity of the sample is through the method in which participants were recruited and the highly segregated neighborhoods (by race, class, and family structure) in which we live. Also, this study is based on narratives of individuals and their acquaintances, who self-select into social support and community groups and therefore are likely to have additional resources that other families may not. In other words, it's likely the mothers who have the extra time and energy to engage in autism community groups and advocacy work also can sit down with me for hours to be interviewed.

I met only two mothers at their place of work who graciously agreed to speak with me during their breaks. The rest I met at their homes, often while their child was in a therapy session in the background, or at coffee shops while their child was watched by a babysitter or at school. Many mothers, who work full-time or multiple jobs and struggle to meet a variety of demands each day, may not have the extra time or bandwidth to engage in regular autism advocacy group work or sit down for hours with a stranger to tell their story. Therefore, the mothers in this book have access to resources—economic, social, and cultural—that reflect their social positions, which in many cases makes it easier (not easy, but easier) for them to access opportunities and autism-related resources that are vital to caregiving, such as high-quality health insurance, education, and language that allow them to advocate for their children effectively in institutional settings, or social networks that grant them access to specialists or top-tier therapists.

For example, some women are financially able to leave their jobs or cut their hours to homeschool their child or transport their child to after-school therapies. In these cases, families can survive and maintain their lifestyle on a single income, a privilege that most American families do not have today. Others have the educational background and language ability that allow them to feel comfortable researching autism providers and therapies or to press for support and accommodations in their child's Individualized Education Plan (IEP) meetings with school authorities. Simply receiving a response in institutional realms is an arduous task for even the most well-resourced caregiver—many families describe many unanswered emails and phone calls and months of missteps in an attempt for just an explanation on how to go about getting an evaluation with the school district, never mind completing the actual evaluation. These are time-consuming, frustrating bureaucratic processes that require persistence, a fight that may just be too much for the many mothers who are just trying to get through their day, keeping everyone clothed, fed, healthy, and safe.

Family socioeconomic status can allow time and flexibility to complete the expert caregiver tasks that are needed to explore, seek out, and secure support for the child. In addition, autism-related services are incredibly expensive (likely not all covered by health insurance) and hard to get. Even with the most comprehensive health insurance, many typical services like speech, occupational therapy, and physical therapy often come with monthlong wait lists and co-pays that add up each month. Families who can afford to *not* wait for in-network services (that come with a lower cost) often turn to private therapies and individualized paid services, such as, private speech therapy, occupational therapy, physical therapy, or applied behavioral analysis therapy (ABA), that can cost hundreds of dollars, each session, out of pocket. In these cases, higher economic status grants greater access to diverse resources and a timelier response. Remember, most of these families have been noting their children's atypical development and exploring neurodiversity and what their children need for years, so being placed on yet another wait list and waiting months for services are something that most families choose to avoid if they can afford it.

The combination of race and class privilege is particularly relevant to understanding experiences in institutional spheres, and especially education and health care. The narratives in this book detail a winding road to the diagnosis, in which mothers feel dismissed and frustrated in clinical interactions where their concerns are not taken seriously by professionals. Based on a wealth of research on bias in health care and advocacy mothering, it is reasonable to assert that more socially disadvantaged mothers, mothers of color, single parents, and low-income mothers may have an even harder time being heard, validated, and supported by doctors and other professionals. This book details many challenges associated with autism caregiving that extends the traditional caregiver role. These challenges, however, are experienced and addressed from a place of relative race and class privilege, which means that low-income families of color, in particular, may experience more obstacles, more waiting, and less support.

Becoming an expert caregiver necessitates a variety of costly resources, including mothers' time and energy. Race and class privilege can make access to these resources just a little bit less arduous or chaotic. Yes, all families, especially with young children, experience many of the same struggles and needs. However, neurodivergent children and children with disabilities and complex and chronic health conditions extend the caregiver role further in ways that typical family and childcare does not. The added deviation from the norm involved in these cases (via disability and health status) translates to additional caregiver responsibilities that are not supported institutionally and are oftentimes undermined socially. This means that families who experience additional forms of social disadvantage, such as families of color and low-income, undocumented, and non–native English-speaking families, experience additional constraints and biases apart of their daily caregiving experience.

Throughout the book, we see the different ways in which mothers make sense of their role as expert caregivers as both a burden and a gift. In almost all cases, the extensive responsibilities and tasks required to meet their children's needs are accepted without protest or questions. Most mothers take on the extended caring role as an assumed part of their role as mothers, and little negotiation with their partners was ever disclosed to me. Mothers do note the times when they felt "unsupported" or "wished everything wasn't on my shoulders," but no one discussed delegating tasks or having their husbands take the lead in the carework for their children. Interrogating the response by partners and men's perspective on carework is a completely different study. The findings would be rich and fascinating; however, it is my choice to ask different questions and to follow in the feminist tradition of foregrounding women's perceptions and experiences in the analysis, as Katherine Allen and Alexis Walker (1992) state: "The purpose is not to exclude men from this analysis, but to place women first."

Therefore, this is a case that furthers the global carework research, in which women take on the lion's share of domestic labor in seemingly natural, assumed, and altruistic ways. The lasting stereotype of women as primary caregivers who oversee the domestic sphere is so entrenched in our society and engrained in family life that the extension of carework into the public sphere (i.e., education, health care, and the community) and the accordant everyday tasks are uncritically pushed into the laps and minds of mothers, without examination. In this way, the intensification of carework and the creation of the expert caregiver can function as a constraining form of gender oppression within the family and outside it. So they, even the mothers who experience race, class, and nuclear family privilege, simultaneously experience disadvantage based on gender. Throughout this book, we see how mothers use carework to work through these nuanced experiences of disadvantage and social exclusion, and to transform their identities and family lives.

Structural Conditions of Autism Carework

Carework is a fascinating concept that sits on the border of many (false) dichotomies and contradictions: it involves love and labor, logic, and emotions. It is paid and unpaid, professional and lay, visible and invisible, and public and private, both a deeply intimate (individual) action and collective social effort. Emily Abel and Margaret Nelson (1990) summarize a key distinction of carework as, "Caregivers are expected to provide love as well as labor" (p. 4). How can we define such a complex sprawling concept and practice? To understand contemporary cases of carework, we must first examine its roots in classical social theory with the naming of reproductive labor as *work* by Marx and Engels, which was later developed by feminists in the Marxist tradition.

Classic social theorists Marx and Engels ([1884] 1972) introduced the idea of "reproductive labor" to capture the traditional domestic tasks of cooking, cleaning, and childrearing that are necessary to maintain and grow a productive labor force. Informal, unpaid reproductive labor in the private sphere is necessary to support workers in the formal, paid public sphere. Further, Marx and Engels situated reproductive labor as key to the successful functioning of a market economy. Therefore, direct links are made between the private and public spheres, and carework is placed firmly within a larger economic framework. In this tradition, more recent feminist scholarship focuses on naming reproductive labor as hard work and examining the ways in which it is socially devalued.

According to sociologist Paula England (2005), the devaluation framework "emphasizes that cultural biases limit both wages and state support for carework because of its association with women.

It addresses the question of why carework has low pay relative to its skill demands" (p. 381). This perspective explains the low pay of feminized occupations and the lack of acknowledgment of unpaid carework as reflections of historical patterns of gender inequality in a patriarchal society. Further, the naturalization of carework as women's work—as work women, in particular, are born to do and "naturally" do better than men—serves as an additional obstacle to naming caring labor as work. Here, there is also an altruistic quality assumed in carework and an intrinsic good associated with being a good caregiver. Carework does not need to be rewarded monetarily if we receive satisfaction and meaning from providing care from the bottom of our hearts. England (1992, 2005) refers to scholarship in this vein that emphasizes the intrinsic rewards associated with carework as the "prisoners of love" framework, which justifies the low pay in caring occupations.

In addition to the focus on caring labor as devalued work with altruistic and intrinsic characteristics, other scholars center the nurturing or relational aspects of carework (Abel & Nelson, 1990; Cancian & Oliker, 2000; Folbre, 2001; Gordon Benner, & Noddings, 1996; Hochschild, 1983, 1995; Tronto, 1993; Tronto & Fisher, 1990). For example, Francesca Cancian and Stacey Oliker (2000) define carework as "feelings of affection and responsibility combined with actions that provide responsively for an individual's personal needs or well-being, in a face-to-face relationship" (p. 2). Sociologist Mignon Duffy (2011) refers to this definition of carework as the "nurturant care perspective," which she delineates in three parts: "First, it focuses on the meeting of personal needs; second, it emphasizes the relational context of care; and finally, it includes not just actions but feelings and emotional responsiveness" (p. 16). The nurturant care perspective draws on an interdisciplinary body of feminist literature in philosophy, economics, political science, history, and psychology, all of which center "sustained, reciprocal emotional connections" (Parks, 2003) between caregiver and recipient as primary in analysis and theorization.

Relationality is what makes carework, whether paid or unpaid, distinct from other types of service work. Caring for children, elders, and disabled people, whether paid or unpaid, is fundamentally intimate and emotional and takes place via everyday one-on-one interactions.

I situated my work within this nurturant framework, as the following chapters illuminate how caregivers meet their children's personal needs within a variety of dynamic relational contexts of care. More broadly, I intend for this work to support the broader feminist call to acknowledge the collective value of care, as a political project and public good, for the betterment of society.

Gender, Carework, and Inequality

Across the globe, women, and especially women of color, complete the majority of carework. Gender is the linchpin to understanding myriad contemporary dynamics of carework, and especially the themes in this case study. As Celia Davies (1995) states, "we need to attend to the cultural content of gender, specifically to the metaphors of masculinity that give a sense of vision and purpose to the public world and that underlie the separation of home and work and inform the notions of bureaucracy and profession" (p. 23). Accordingly, first this section highlights key contributions on gender, unpaid carework, and motherhood.

All the primary caregivers in this study are women and mothers, and that is not a coincidence or an anomaly. An extensive body of literature documents the unequal, unpaid, and gendered nature of household labor, and especially regarding childcare. The entrenched structure of gender in society allocates women to the private, domestic, caring sphere and men to the public sphere of economic breadwinning, institutional engagement, and paid labor. However, scholarship on contemporary motherhood also points out that the lines are more blurred for economically disadvantaged women and women of color for whom constructions of motherhood also include breadwinning, mostly due to necessity (Thornton Dill, 1994; Armenia, 2009; Glenn, 1992 Jarrett & Jefferson, 2003).

Feminist approaches to informal family carework, or maternal caregiving, in the family are of particular relevance to this study. Critical feminist approaches all challenge this belief that women's "natural" role is in the home and in charge of the domestic sphere, as Marjorie DeVault (1991) summarizes: "It is an argument that is fundamentally about women's 'place' in family life, rather than about identity, an argument that aims to show how women are continually recruited—whatever their psychological predispositions—into participation in social relations that produce their subordination" (p. 13). Accordingly, the chapters that follow describe paradoxical ways that expert caregiving can push women into "social relations that produce their subordination" (DeVault, 1991, p. 13) and at the same time can subvert traditional gender norms and gendered power dynamics in various social institutions.

The Intensification of Family Carework: Caring for Disabled Children and Medicalization

As described by DeVault above, more recent feminist scholarship on maternal caregiving that operates at the level of social organization (Lareau, 2011; Christopher, 2012; Blum, 2015; Brenton, 2017) builds on Sharon Hays's (1996) idea of "intensive mothering," which is "child-centered, expert-guided, emotionally absorbing, labor-intensive and financially expensive." "Intensive mothering" captures the increasing pressures put on mothers to expend exorbitant resources (i.e., time, energy, emotions, money, etc.) on raising their children while following the latest "expert" advice. Here, the child's needs are placed above all else and often come at the expense of the mother's interests and well-being. The pressures, and the stakes, are incredibly high for mothers to "do the right thing" and set up their children to succeed in an increasingly competitive global world. The mothers in the following chapters push the bounds of intensive mothering even further by taking on a variety of professional skills and extending their carework outside the home and into public organizational and institutional spheres. Further, the expansion of good mothering is embedded in power relations and can be a source for perpetuating inequalities. This study builds on this body of work and shows how caring for disabled children significantly extends the expectations, roles, and practices associated with good mothering and maternal carework.

Many gender scholars have written on the intensification of carework involved in caring for disabled children with emphasis on securing educational and medical resources (Litt, 2004; Blum, 2007; Malacrida, 2003, 2004). Jacquelyn Litt (2004) refers to the extension of carework outside the home as "advocacy care work," "a type of caring activity that women described as going beyond the typical work of linking family services to other institutions" (p. 628). Similarly, sociologist Linda Blum (2007, 2015) describes these exemplar women as "vigilantes" who are situated in opposition to medical and educational authority; vigilantes "seize authority against adversaries who are its legitimate holders" (p. 206). In the vein of Litt's (2004) and Blum's (2007) research, feminist scholars provide additional insight into "mother-blame" experiences in the medicalization of atypical children's behaviors and how mothers assert their agency especially raising children with ADHD (Malacrida, 2003, 2004; Singh, 2004). For example, Singh (2004) shows how mothers are blamed not just for their child's "bad behavior" but also for giving their ADHD children a "quick fix" with Ritalin. In this way, child neurodivergent behaviors are associated with poor parenting and "bad mothering." These scholars analyze the different ways in which mothers are blamed for their children's disruptive behaviors and how the jurisdiction of medicine expands far beyond the clinic or doctor-patient interactions.

Together, these studies demonstrate the impacts associated with dominant constructions of disability and neurodivergence as "bad," "deviant," and a "problem" for which mothers, in particular, are at fault—literally to blame. This harmful construction reflects a deep lack of understanding about disability and neurodivergence and a system of social arrangements that are founded on and uphold ableist principles. Simply put, assumptions and expectations that discriminate against disabled and neurodivergent people are entrenched in cultural ideas and norms about motherhood and family.

Each chapter shows how lay caregivers shape and challenge mainstream institutional practices and social discourses about autism through their everyday life experiences on playgrounds, at grocery stores, and in schools and doctor's offices. Interestingly, while fighting for a diagnosis, caregivers become active agents in the medicalization of their children's behaviors while also challenging the traditional cultural authority of medicine and hierarchical doctor-patient interactions. Therefore, carework can be a powerful agent of both medicalization and demedicalization, which provides a nuanced contribution to the literature on carework, motherhood, and medicalization. At the same time, I highlight how this community is constrained by structural forces (insufficient care systems), internal community divisions, and caregiver fears and preferences. In this vein, the following chapters show how unpaid family carework can push the boundaries of public and private life and normative ideas of ability and good mothering, all through the process of becoming an expert caregiver.

Caregivers' Stories

The chapters in this book are organized with the intent to expand in scope and scale from the most intimate unit of self-identity to meso-level family and community-based dynamics, and lastly, to macro-oriented public advocacy and social reform efforts. Together, these chapters link individual, interactional, and institutional dynamics associated with expert caregiving.

Chapter 1 provides an overview of the complex backdrop that informs contemporary autism carework in the United States and includes a brief history that highlights key shifts in the professional construction and diagnostic criteria for autism. Importantly, this chapter also unpacks the two primary models for understanding autism today, the Biomedical Model and the Social Model of Disability (including Neurodiversity), and the tensions between these primary frameworks for understanding autism in the United States today.

Then, firmly located on the micro level, chapter 2 details the birth of the expert caregiver, and specifically the root causes that spark transformation in caregivers' ideas of themselves, motherhood and family, and autism. This chapter foregrounds the important relational process in which caregiver self-identity is ruptured and later repaired within the caring experience. Thus, this chapter functions as the first step in a larger story of how autism caregivers become experts, and the complex and relational reasons for why they do.

Chapter 3 builds on the previous chapter by describing the process through which carework activities intensify to include taking on a variety of professional roles and skill sets, which become a part of the expert caregiver toolkit. The jurisdiction of unpaid informal carework expands past traditional in-home carework boundaries through engagement with medical diagnostics, scientific research and literature, teaching and lesson planning, skilled nursing, and specialized knowledge and modalities specific to support therapies (i.e., PT, OT, speech therapy, and diet and nutrition) with what feels like life-and-death consequences. As a result, sophisticated expert caregivers emerge who are highly educated on autism and able to engage in medical jargon and specialized discussions with diverse professionals, navigate institutional bureaucracies, and act as multiple therapists, all while advocating for their children and caring for their families.

Chapter 4 begins to shift attention off the micro level and details the ways in which expert caregiving is marked by the extension of caring labor outside one's private home and individual family and into the surrounding local community. Here, expert caregiving becomes a public, prosocial practice, through which caregivers operate at organizational and institutional levels.

Then, chapter 5 maximizes chapter 4's conceptualization of community carework to show the transformative potential of carework to engage with institutions to promote structural change. Additionally, key factors that constrain the practice of expert carework as a transformative public project are identified, which include private versus public models for understanding, the "double-edged sword" of medicalization, and pragmatic concerns associated with resource loss. Together, chapters 4 and 5 conceptualize a distinction of expert caregiving, which is the participation in community carework activities that bridge false dichotomies of public and private, individual and society, and lay and professional.

Finally, chapter 6 highlights the ways this analysis reveals paradoxical lessons for scholarly discussion on carework, gender, family, and medicalization and lessons gleaned for the transformative power of carework. Finally, in the tradition of the feminist ethic of care, I reiterate how carework is a deeply personal practice that holds significant societal impact and why carework and expert caregivers deserve to be valued and visible.

Throughout the chapters in this book, you'll see how the expert caregiver is one person who faces unbelievably daunting tasks of filling or reforming persistent institutional gaps, primarily in education and health care, and subverting bias cultural norms. Without institutional support, answers to their questions, or pragmatic avenues to access resources, lay caregivers become the experts. Their trials and tribulations, especially when navigating the boundaries of professional/lay and public/private worlds, illuminate a type of carework that is increasingly relevant to a growing number of young families caring for neurodivergent, disabled, medically fragile, and/or chronically ill children. These stories offer a vivid picture of the contemporary realities of caring for autistic children, and in doing so, further empirical case studies on informal nurturant carework and caregiving for disabled and neurodivergent children. By voicing the stories in this book, I hope to spotlight these families and reveal the oft-invisible complex challenges that drive them to become expert caregivers in the first place.

"Becoming" is a strategic choice to capture how this process is not linear or fixed and is fundamentally relational. In other words, expert caregiving is shaped by the broader social world, and especially vis-à-vis structural flaws in health care, education, gender and family, and disability. Accordingly, the title of this book signals the fluid process inherent in expert caregiving today, which occurs within a paltry U.S. social safety net and private orientation toward care and disability that render attention to both—carework and disability—invisible.

Note: Identity-first language is used in this book, as opposed to person-first language, per the preference of the autistic community.

1
Autism Complexities
Competing Paradigms and Historical Context

As I sit at the kitchen table with Serena, a mother of two autistic children ages six and nine, she gives me a sly look and says, "Listen to this one." My interest was piqued, and she proceeded to tell a little story: "When I was driving down to LA for my uncle's funeral, I heard an advertisement for a fundraiser to cure autism that my local Kia dealership was putting on. You know, one of these 'We need money to fund the latest study to cure Autism' thing. I was so angry when I heard that. I was like, 'Cure?' So, I pulled over and I called the Kia dealership. I called the freaking dealership! I'm talking to the receptionist, and I say, 'I'm going to be really calm with you because this is not you, but I'd like to know who did that commercial about curing autism, because I need to talk to that person to educate them. You don't cure autism. It's not a disease.'"

I could hear the anger in her voice and the passion. She felt it was so important to tell me this story, so I asked her, "What does the word 'disease' bring out? Can you speak to that?" She replied, "I think it's because it makes it seem like it's something so sad or bad. You know, when somebody has breast cancer, it's like, 'Oh, my God, I'm so sorry, that is just terrible.' I'm not sorry that my kids have autism; it's not a terrible sad thing! They're not fighting for their lives. It's just . . . It's part of who they are. I'm dyslexic.

That's how I read. That's how I see things. It's just how I decode things; it's who I am. That's how I wish other people would understand autism and my kiddos."

This chapter serves to provide a basic understanding of the complex backdrop that informs contemporary autism carework in the United States and begins with a history that highlights key shifts in understanding and the clinical criteria for the autism diagnosis.

Major Historical Shifts in Diagnostic Classification and Criteria

The tensions that surround autism today are similarly found throughout the history of the diagnosis. Cultural context and dominant academic and lay popular discourse play a fundamental role in the past and present construction and interpretation of autism.

The history of the autism diagnosis begins in 1911, when German psychiatrist Eugen Bleuler used the term "autism" to describe a symptom associated with severe cases of childhood schizophrenia. According to Bleuler (1911), in the vein of Freudian psychoanalytics, autistic thinking was characterized by "infantile wishes to avoid unsatisfying realities and replace them with fantasies and hallucinations." Autism continued to be conceptualized in direct relationship to childhood schizophrenia throughout the 1950s and 1960s by psychiatrists and psychologists in Britain and the United States.

Moreover, in 1943, autism as an official diagnosis was mentioned by Dr. Leo Kanner, a child psychologist, in a paper on a case study of eleven children who shared a set of puzzling symptoms: the need for solitude and sameness (Kanner, 1943). Kanner's (1943) paper also supported a biological explanation for autism, as he states, "We must, then, assume that these children have come into the world with innate inability to form the usual, biologically provided affective contact with people, just as other children come into the world with innate physical or intellectual handicaps" (p. 220).

However, in his 1949 follow-up paper, Kanner shifted away from a biological explanation to a psychological explanation, which emphasized the role of poor parenting and parental personality as the fundamental factors that explain childhood autism. The shift to parent-blame and psychological explanations is argued to be highly reflective of the psychoanalytic turn in American culture in the late 1940s and early 1950s (Grandin & Panek, 2013).

More specifically, Kanner's 1949 paper introduced the idea of the cold, uncaring "refrigerator mother" as a leading cause for autism, which was further circulated by Bruno For those with autism predisposition, both Kanner (1949) and Bettelheim (1967) promoted the idea that poor parenting, particularly by cold, emotionally distant mothers, was the trigger for autistic behaviors in childhood; an argument that has been repeatedly refuted in the literature. Importantly, Margaret Gibson and Patty Douglas (2018) point out that the scientific history of autism is inherently social and unequal: "The children who became the basis for Kanner's [1943] descriptions of early childhood autism as a distinct if rare disorder were overwhelmingly white and male, with unusually well-educated, middle-class parents who were themselves university professors or doctors. The educational and professional achievements of the early patients' fathers and (in a more muted and ambivalent tone) their mothers were front and centre in the early case studies, and in much of the writing on autism throughout the twentieth century" (p. 7).

Gibson and Douglas (2018) persuasively articulate the distinctly *social* (as opposed to biological) roots of *biomedical* understandings of autism, in which autistic behaviors are deemed deviant: "Importantly, then, from its inception, autism has been a way to describe what one could call surprising deviants; that is, autism emerged as a marker of children who did not fit pre-existing categories of the 'unfit'" (p. 7).

Meanwhile, autism remained excluded from official classification in the American Psychiatric Association's *Diagnostic and Statistical Manual of Mental Disorders* (*DSM*) until the 1980s. Beginning with the first publication of the *DSM-I* in 1952, autism was mentioned only in relation to schizophrenia. For example, in describing "schizophrenic reaction," it states, "Psychotic reactions in [a] child, manifesting primarily autism," with no further explanation or definition of what "autism" means. Similarly, in the second publication of the *DSM-II* in 1968, there was minimal use of the word "autism" to describe symptoms related to schizophrenia (e.g., "autistic, atypical, and withdrawn behavior"). Therefore, early research and theoretical discussions on autism are deeply rooted in cultural and intellectual discourses of the time. Here, autism is conceptualized as a form or symptom of childhood schizophrenia and is grounded heavily in temporally specific mother-blame cultural discourses.

Later, in 1980, the *DSM-III* decoupled autism from schizophrenia and brought back biological arguments about brain development into discussions of autism. The *DSM-III* lists "infantile autism" or "Kanner's Syndrome" under the broader diagnostic category of Pervasive Developmental Disorders (PDD). The infantile autism diagnosis required six criteria: (1) onset before thirty months, (2) pervasive lack of responsiveness to other people, (3) gross deficits in language development, (4) if speech is present, peculiar speech patterns, such as immediate and delayed echolalia, metaphorical language, pronominal reversal, (5) bizarre responses to various aspects of the environment (e.g., resistance to change, peculiar interest in or attachments to animate or inanimate objects), and (6) the absence of schizophrenia (APA, 1980). In 1987, the *DSM-III-R* expanded the diagnostic criteria for autism from six to sixteen and included a name change from "infantile autism" to "autistic disorder." The drastic expansion of the "autistic disorder" criteria in the *DSM-III* led to higher rates of diagnosis. However, they remain much lower in comparison to current autism rates in 2023. For context, in the 1980s, U.S. autism prevalence was reported as 1 in 10,000; in the 1990s, prevalence was 1 in 2,500; and today, autism rates stand at 1 in 36 (CDC, 2023).

While Kanner was introducing the idea of autism in the 1940s, Hans Asperger (1944), an Austrian pediatrician, identified "autistic psychopathy" to denote a category of children who shared the following behaviors: "a lack of empathy, little ability to form friendships, one-sided conversations, intense absorption in a special interest, and clumsy movements." Asperger's findings were popularized by British psychiatrist and parent of an autistic child Lorna Wing (Wing, 1981), which were later formalized into an official diagnosis called Asperger's syndrome (or Asperger's) in 1994 in the *DSM-IV.* Here, Asperger's was categorized based on the following key criteria: (1) qualitative impairment in social interaction and (2) restricted repetitive and stereotyped patterns of behavior, interests, and activities (APA, 1994). Symptoms also must fall outside the criteria for PDD and schizophrenia. Historically, what distinguished Asperger's syndrome from autism was the lack of clinically significant speech and language delays or cognitive delays (most children diagnosed with Asperger's were both speech and cognitively typical).

Most importantly, the addition of Asperger's syndrome to the *DSM-IV* was a significant move in the reframing of autism as more of a *spectrum*, as opposed to a singular black-and-white diagnosis. However, in 2013, Asperger's syndrome was eliminated from the *DSM-V* and replaced with autism spectrum disorder, due to research showing inconsistency in the ways in which Asperger's and PDD diagnoses were applied. Therefore, according to the *DSM-V,* individuals who previously fit the Asperger's criteria could be evaluated for the newly reorganized autism spectrum disorder or a new category called social and communication disorder (SCD), which is further explained in the following section.

Current Diagnostic Classification: Autism Spectrum Disorder (ASD)

According to the most recent *DSM-V-TR* guidelines, an autism diagnosis requires "persistent deficits in each of three areas of social communication and interaction (e.g., abnormal social approach and failure of back-and-forth conversation, total lack of facial expressions and nonverbal communication), plus at least two of the four types of restricted, repetitive behaviors (e.g., repetitive motor movements, echolalia, and ritualized patterns of verbal or nonverbal behavior)" (APA, 2022). Clinical diagnosis requires that symptoms are present in early development, but symptoms "may not become fully manifest until social demands exceed limited capacities or may be masked by learned strategies in later life" (APA, 2022).

It is important to note that a few years previously, in 2013, the *DSM-V* (APA, 2013) collapsed all previous subdisorders associated with the autism spectrum, such as autistic disorder, Asperger's syndrome, pervasive developmental disorder, and childhood disintegrative disorder, into one category that is now called autism spectrum disorder. In doing so, the current autism diagnosis emphasizes severity levels more so than in the past *DSM* versions. For example, "individuals who have marked deficits in social communication, but whose symptoms do not otherwise meet criteria for autism spectrum disorder" are recommended to be evaluated for a separate new disorder called social (pragmatic) communication disorder. It is believed that most individuals previously diagnosed with Asperger's will meet social communication disorder criteria.

The recent shifts in the reclassification of autism in the *DSM* come with some tensions and concerns in both the professional and lay autistic community. The professional majority position is that these changes will not have a negative impact on individuals but are designed to keep diagnostic thresholds high. To date, there are not yet conclusive data on the exact outcomes of these diagnostic changes on overall U.S. prevalence rates and access to services for children and families.

Competing Paradigms for Understanding Autism Today

The history presented above both reflects and informs the two primary paradigms for understanding autism today in the United States. The next important contextual piece of the story is to understand that the *DSM* reflects the dominant biomedical model of autism, which is largely in conflict with the social model of disability and neurodiversity framework of autism. These paradigms—the biomedical model and the social model of disability and neurodiversity—provide two competing worldviews or maps for understanding autism today in the United States, which I now turn to unpack.

THE BIOMEDICAL MODEL

As detailed above, the biomedical model of autism defines autism as a bioneurological developmental disorder that varies in severity, though it is characterized by persistent deficits in social communication, and repetitive patterns of behavior, interests, or activities (APA, 2022). It is not a single disorder, which accounts for the range or spectrum of traits and behaviors. Autism is characterized in varying degrees by difficulties in social interaction, verbal and nonverbal communication, repetitive behaviors like hand flapping, and "special interests" or an intense focus on a chosen topic. Autistic children can show a variety of special traits or hypersensitivities to stimuli (i.e., sound, touch, tastes, smells, and light), sleep disturbances, and gastrointestinal (GI) disturbances. All these present differently, if at all, and range in severity from one child to another.

What is more, comorbidity is frequent with diagnoses such as attention deficit hyperactivity disorder (ADHD), bipolar disorder, obsessive compulsive disorder, depression, and anxiety. Twenty-five percent of children in this research study were diagnosed with both autism and ADHD, and one child was diagnosed with autism, ADHD, and bipolar disorder. Almost all parents reported consistent challenges with hypersensitivities, such as picky eating (a sensory processing–related issue), speech delays if verbal, gastrointestinal issues, and sleep disturbances.

Medically, autism is a disorder of the individual brain, though unlike ADHD or depression it cannot be treated via psychotherapy or psychiatric drugs alone. Autism appears to have its roots in very early brain development, though no single cause or explanation has been found. To date, the biomedical causes of autism are widely contested, though theories primarily center on genetics, environmental exposure, childhood vaccine injury, and allostatic load (Trottier, Srivastava, & Walker, 1999; Persico & Bourgeron,

2006; Freitag, 2007; Happé & Plomin, 2006; Gershwind, 2009; Herbert et al., 2006; Herbert, 2010). As Jennifer Singh (2016) investigates in her book *Multiple Autisms*, the search for an "autism gene," or set of genes, is a billion-dollar industry, and a "major funding priority in the United States" (p. 4). Yet, the "autism gene" has not been found, and currently, there exists no definitive etiology, "cure," or exact treatment plan. As Singh states (2016), "It is estimated that approximately 20–25 percent of autism cases are a result of known genetic mechanisms, leaving the cause of 75–80 percent of cases unknown" (p. 4). The lack of a singular definitive cause, biomarker, or etiology of autism heightens the anxieties felt by caregivers, especially early on in their journeys.

Autism Interventions: Biomedical. In this model, normative modalities to treat autistic symptoms in children include speech therapy, occupational therapy, physical therapy, FDA-approved medications (i.e., antipsychotic drugs like Risperidone and Aripiprazole to improve moods and behaviors), and a variety of behavioral therapy programs, notably Applied Behavioral Analysis (ABA), which is the longest-standing biomedical treatment for autistic children.

Applied behavior analysis works to change a child's nonnormative and dangerous behaviors using positive reinforcement learning principles derived from B. F. Skinner's work in behavioral psychology. Starting in the 1960s as a part of the Young Autism Project clinic at UCLA, psychologist Ole Ivar Lovaas used behaviorist strategies to teach autistic children normative social skills, address language and cognitive delays, and decrease problematic behaviors to avoid institutionalization (Lovaas, Schaeffer, & Simmons, 1965; Lovaas, Berberich, Perloff, & Schaeffer, 1966). Behaviorist strategies intend to cultivate compliance in children by using operant conditioning methods that reward desired behaviors and punish undesirable ones.

More recently, "new ABA" programs build on the Lovaas Method to combine early-intervention principles with behavior analysis in a play-based and more child-friendly delivery model to reach children as young as twelve months. Most ABA programs are used with children between the ages of two and eight and can last months to years (Gibson, Pritchard, & de Lemos, 2021).

Research supports that early intervention ABA therapies are an effective treatment modality for minimizing severity of autistic behavioral symptoms in verbal children (DeMyer, Hingtgen, & Jackson 1981; Lovaas, 1987; McEachin, Smith, & Lovaas, 1993; Sallows & Graupner, 2005; Cohen, Amerine-Dickens, & Smith, 2006) and are endorsed by multiple organizations (e.g., the United States Surgeon General, National Institute of Mental Health, and the American Psychological Association).

More recent follow-up studies on ABA efficacy, specifically based on the Lovaas and Early Start Denver Models, conclude that early intensive behavioral therapy (EIBI) is an efficient method to improve intellectual functioning and adaptive behavior, such as communication, daily living, and socialization in young autistic children (Eikeseth, 2009; Eldevik, Jahr, & Smith 2006; Eldevik, Hastings, Jahr, & Hughes, 2012; Rogers & Vismara, 2008). However, the idea of "autism recovery" and ABA methods of any kind are highly controversial and profoundly refuted by many autistic adults and advocates, parents, and professionals working in the field. Instead, critics of ABA support neurodiversity-affirming interventions in alignment with the social model of disability.

THE SOCIAL MODEL OF DISABILITY

In opposition to the medical model's emphasis on individual deficits or bodily impairments that need to be fixed or cured via medical interventions, the social model of disability defines autism as a neurotype that functions as a category of disability and identity. A neurotype is one individual form of brain wiring, or how different parts of our brains connect with or "speak to each other." Autistic brains are wired differently from neurotypical brains; neuroimaging studies find clear differences in the structural and functional brain development in autistic children and adults.[1] Autistic brain wiring is referred to as neurodivergent, and typical

---

1. See Ha, Sohn, Kim, Sim, & Cheon (2015).

brain development and cognitive function are referred to as neurotypical. As a result of different brain wiring, neurodivergent individuals often communicate, think, behave, and learn differently from neurotypical assumptions and expectations in these areas; they are different, not broken, or wrong.

Simply put, autistic brains look and function differently from neurotypical brains from childhood through adulthood, which informs the physical or identifiable differences in social behaviors and traits. Due to different brain wiring, autistic people can have sensitivities to things that neurotypicals do not and often take for granted, such as having back-and-forth verbal conversations and overstimulation from loud noises, smells, or sensations on the body like tags in clothes that cause dysregulation. These sensory sensitivities are common in autistic children, though they are often misunderstood by neurotypical people who may not be able to see, hear, smell, or feel the trigger. Further, when children are over- or understimulated and become dysregulated, their behaviors are often judged as "naughty," "lacking discipline," and the result of "bad parenting," which become sources of social marginalization and shame for caregivers. On the other hand, autistics are known to have "spiky profiles," which means there are a variety of strengths associated with neurodivergent neurology like superior ability to think outside the box and be creative, hyperfocus on details, and have exceptional long-term memory.

From a social model of disability perspective, disability does not emerge from a defect in an individual's body or mind, but instead from societal restrictions that limit an individual to participate fully in life. More specifically, in 1976, the Union of the Physically Impaired Against Segregation (UPIAS) defined disability as "the disadvantage or restriction of activity caused by a contemporary social organization which takes no or little account of people who have physical impairments and thus excludes them from the mainstream of social activities" (p. 14). Later, this definition was extended to also include intellectual, mental, and sensory impairments. Michael Oliver (1990), a principal theorist of the social model of disability, conceptualized this model as a way to think differently about disability, away from the individual body and from outside the realm of medicine. Accordingly, disability is defined as a collective experience that is fundamentally produced by external social arrangements and the built world.

Disability scholar Carol Thomas (2004) articulates the significance of this social model for understanding disability: "Disability now resided in a nexus of social relationships connecting those socially identified as impaired and those deemed non-impaired or 'normal,' relationships that worked to exclude and disadvantage the former while promoting the relative inclusion and privileging of the latter" (p. 33). Thomas (2004a) further clarifies, "Disability is social exclusion on the grounds of impairment. Impairment does not cause disability, certainly not, but it is the raw material upon which disability works" (p. 42). Accordingly, it is not the autistic brain or neurotype but the social arrangements within society that create the disabling conditions. In other words, autism is not intrinsically disabling; rather, being autistic in a neurotypical social world creates experiences of social exclusion and collective oppression. As Vic Finkelstein (2001a) states, "Disability is something imposed on top of our impairments by the way we are unnecessarily isolated and excluded from full participation in society. Disabled people are therefore an oppressed group in society." The normative and taken-for-granted ways in which society is organized and people's neurotypical assumptions for social behavior create the conditions for which autism can operate as a disability.

Since the mid-1970s, there have been much debate and critique within disability studies on the social model of disability, which is beyond the scope of this study but addressed well by Oliver (2013), who reiterates the central objective in the social model: "I have never seen the social model as anything more than a tool to improve peoples' lives and I have been happy to agree that it does not do many of the things its opponents criticize it for not doing. Indeed, in 1990 I published a book that attempted to develop a more all-encompassing explanation of what was happening to disabled people in the modern world" (p. 1025). Following Carol Thomas's (2004) call to develop the social-relational aspect in the social model, this study illuminates different social relationships that inform experiences of exclusion in public and private spheres, and later, how these lessons are translated in the process of becoming an agentic expert caregiver.

THE NEURODIVERSITY FRAMEWORK

Interrogating "normality" and neurotypical cultural norms is at the heart of the neurodiversity approach. "Neurodiversity" was coined by autistic sociologist Judy Singer in 1998, in which she carved out a new category of disability and political engagement, which focuses singularly on brain differences. Through this lens, neurological differences, like autism, dyslexia, and ADHD, occur naturally and have a range of strengths associated with them (as opposed to an emphasis on deficits). Rooted in the social model of disability and informed by the disability rights movement, the neurodiversity framework understands autism as an integral aspect of one's core identity, like our gender, race, and class. Additionally, the neurodiversity movement "is led by autistic self-advocates fighting for autism acceptance" (Hughes, 2016). Importantly, Singer's (1998, 1999, 2016) conceptualization of neurodiversity intended to operate more as a middle-ground approach that bridged oversimplified emphasis on the biological body (medical model) *or* society (social model) in definitions of disability, "to transcend the construction of binary oppositions such as 'Medical Model vs. Social Model'" (p. 555).

More recently, disability studies scholars like Anna Stenning and Hanna Bertilsdotter-Rosqvist (2021) have put forth a new critical paradigm on neurodiversity, which focuses on the cultural construction of normality that aims for "greater recognition, representation and resources for those at the neurological margins of academic discourse" (p. 1534). Here, the neurodiversity framework for understanding autism asks us to think seriously about who and what are defined as "normal" or "typical," and the subjectivity of the autism diagnosis. Currently, there are no biomarkers or genetic tests that can diagnose or definitively confirm autism. The medical diagnosis of autism (and many other neurodivergent conditions) is based on a medical practitioner's interpretation of atypical behaviors observed in isolated clinic visits (and other contrived settings) and parental survey results. Therefore, the neurodiversity framework calls attention to the questionable evidence-based diagnostic practices and room for bias in understanding normality, deviance, and the resulting medicalization of "atypical" behaviors.

Simply put, from a neurodiversity perspective, there is nothing deficient or problematic about the autistic brain; it is simply different and a natural part of human diversity. This model asks us to question how our inherent assumptions about the ways in which our everyday lives operate may uphold systemic barriers and bias expectations against those who were born with different neurology.

Autism Interventions: Social Model of Disability and Neurodiversity-Affirming Interventions. Neurodiversity-affirming interventions embrace the uniqueness and strengths of autistic children and aim to support skill-building, self-advocacy, body autonomy, and independence. As opposed to a central focus on correcting or hiding dysfunctions and deficits, neurodiversity-affirming interventions aim to empower individuals by building on their existing strengths and interests through supportive therapies and access to resources. Specifically, accommodations and resources for children and adults in this vein include supporting an individual's particular sensory needs through providing noise-canceling headphones or earplugs, weighted blankets, movement breaks, and sensory diets to identify triggers and promote emotional and body regulation, increasing accessibility of augmentative or alternative communication (AAC) devices, and access to strengths-based neurodivergent-affirming therapies, like speech-language therapy, occupational therapy, equine therapy, physical therapy, and counseling that help children build important communication, physical, and social-emotional skills to increase well-being and gain independence.

Additionally, supporting neurodiversity in the K–12 classroom includes accommodations such as student access to fidget toys and voice-to-text digital resources, integration of visual schedules, graphic organizers, and visual or written, rather than auditory, instructions into the classroom. Such accommodations recognize some of the common challenges that neurodivergent students have in the classroom and make important changes to allow them to thrive. Importantly, the social model of disability and neurodiversity framework call for broader cultural change to challenge the social construction of "normality" and "abnormality"—to think differently about difference—to allow all people the agency to move through the world safely (without harm) and with community, health, and loving care.

Accordingly, these interventions stand in direct opposition to the biomedical model's emphasis on ABA. The controversy that surrounds ABA is centered on its operant conditioning methods that are designed to increase compliance and change autistic behavior to match neurotypical norms and expectations. For example, Laura Anderson's (2023) recent qualitative research with autistic adults who received ABA as a child found risks of harm associated with ABA:

> Overwhelmingly, the largest implication for the practice of ABA is that there is a risk of genuine long-term harm to people who receive ABA. For some of the participants, that harm was simply being misunderstood. For other participants, being misunderstood was only part of the problem; the other part of the problem was that they felt like the interventions and demands were counter to a core aspect of who they are as a person. They felt dehumanized, traumatized, and abused by the therapy they received. As a result, they suffer long-term mental health challenges and feel like they are required to mask, or hide who they are (p. 14).

Similarly, Owen McGill and Anna Robinson (2021) interviewed ten autistic adults who received ABA as children, who expressed negative impacts associated with ABA: "The majority of participants' reflections (n=7) referred to being left with feelings of self-rejection and a sense of self-loathing as a consequence of their experience of ABA." Additionally, this study highlights the connection between ABA's compliance training and increased vulnerability to abuse by authority figures, in which respondents noted that ABA methods "made it harder for me to say no to people who hurt me later." Similarly, operant conditioning methods at the core of ABA can lead to problematic levels of compliance, low intrinsic motivation, and lack of independent functioning later in adulthood for autistic adults (Carr, 1977; Minshawi et al., 2014; Weiss, 2003).

Additionally, both lay autistics and academic researchers have identified troubling links between ABA's founder Lovaas's goal to change autistic children's "deviant" behaviors and gender-shaping behaviorism. In other words, Lovaas's body of work demonstrates an interest in using behaviorism to shape nonconforming bodies and minds to meet dominant ideals of normality. As Gibson and Douglas (2018) write, "Less commonly recognized is Lovaas's simultaneous involvement in the Feminine Boy Project during the 1970s, where he catalogued and developed interventions into the gender and sexual non-conforming identities and behaviors of young people" (McGuire, 2016; Silberman, 2015; Yergeau, 2018). Accordingly, Gibson and Douglas (2018) present compelling evidence that supports lay anecdotes and nonacademic sources that problematize the roots of ABA.

Therefore, it is evident that significant controversy remains in both lay and professional best practices for ways to address autistic symptoms and maximize the well-being for autistic individuals. Relevant to this study, these tensions complicate the social caring experience, in which caregivers are simply trying to do what is best for their children and what is "best" is contested and unclear. Throughout the chapters in this book, caregivers show how medical uncertainty, gaps in health care, and mixed messages translate into the real lives of American families and the social caring experience.

SOCIOLOGY OF CHRONIC ILLNESS AND DISABILITY

Medical sociologists who study health and illness present a different orientation toward disability that contrasts with the social model in disability scholarship. Whereas disability scholars center oppression in the definition and experience of disability, medical sociologists understand disability as caused by illness or impairment and involving some degree of social disadvantage and dependency (e.g., collective experience of oppression is not foregrounded). The emphasis on structural analysis and group oppression inherent in the social model of disability is a point of disagreement or critique with medical sociologists who study chronic illness and disability. Tom Shakespeare and Nicholas Watson (2001) describe the nuanced relationship between impairment and disability that underlies the tension between disability scholars' and medical sociologist's approaches to disability: Impairment and disability are not dichotomous, but describe different places on a continuum, or different aspects of a single experience. It is difficult to determine where impairment ends and disability starts, but such vagueness need not be debilitating. Disability is a complex dialectic of biological, psychological, cultural and socio-political factors, which cannot be extricated except with imprecision" (p. 22).

Most notably, medical sociologists and anthropologists use a chronic illness narrative approach to make sense of and to give meaning to unique experiences of suffering (Kleinman, 1988; Frank, 1995; Tanner, 1999; B. Good, 1994; Good & Good, 2000; Charmaz, 2000; Mattingly & Garro, 2000; Mattingly, 1994, 2012; Williams, 2000). This wealth of research on narrative, illness, and identity was largely prompted by Elliott Mishler's (1984) concept of the "voice of the lifeworld" and Arthur Kleinman's (1988) interpretive paradigm for the study of clinical narratives. This "narrative turn" in medicine has led to increased interdisciplinary awareness of the importance of privileging patient voices and placing illness within a larger social and cultural context.

Arthur Frank (1995), in his seminal work *The Wounded Storyteller*, describes culturally specific forms of narrative, or general storylines, that authors use to organize their illness experiences and to explain them to others, which are useful in describing and analyzing the life stories told in this case. Recent case studies have applied Frank's narrative typologies to help make sense of living with HIV (Ezzy, 2000), breast cancer (Thomas-Maclean, 2004), and chronic fatigue syndrome (Whitehead, 2006), all which center power and control on patients instead of on medical authorities. Australian sociologist David Gray has written extensively on how narrative can create coherence in families with autistic children (2001) and parental psychosocial well-being and experiences associated with stigma (1993, 2002, 2003).

Disability scholars have critiqued the overly individualistic emphasis in illness narrative scholarship as disconnected from the broader structural context that gives rise to disability. However, studies by medical sociologists like Kathy Charmaz (2020) challenge this critique by bridging the gap between the individual and society. For example, in her work on the disabling conditions associated with chronic illness, Charmaz (2020) situates very personal experiences of suffering and stigma within a much larger neoliberal context, thereby foregrounding the role of structural arrangements in the creation of disability. In this tradition, I see narrative as a useful way to provide insight into how patients and caregivers construct and order their experiences and reality, within the existing paltry structural contexts of care. Therefore, individual experience, cultural knowledge, and institutional context are inextricably linked.

Other medical sociologists like Michael Bury (2000) argue for a middle ground between the social model of disability that foregrounds structural arrangements and oppression and Frank's agentic, overly individualistic "wounded storyteller" paradigm: "The mid-range, between a wounded storyteller and an overly politicized conception would, as [Irving] Zola suggests, seem to offer the best way forward" (p. 182). I seek to exist here in the middle ground by highlighting the utility of individual narratives for a rich and complicated discussion of the high stakes and deeply personal experiences involved in the autism caring experience, also contextualized within a system of structural constraints and relational experiences of exclusion.

In sum, this chapter serves to paint a nuanced and complex backdrop for the empirical findings that are to come in the following chapters. Throughout the history of autism, key shifts in lay understanding and professional classification of autistic symptoms are informed by existing social and cultural norms. Further, the ways in which we understand, classify, and treat autism today remain in flux. The complexities associated with understanding autism are reflected in the tensions among the two competing paradigms that provide fundamentally different orientations to autism today. How we understand and classify autism matters because each paradigm has unique objectives and approaches that guide best practices for interventions and support for the autistic community, their families, and society. Now, with this broader contextual picture in mind, I turn to center the fifty caregivers and their families who share their stories on becoming expert caregivers.

2
Tracing Transformation
The Birth of the Expert Caregiver

After a relaxing drive on hilly country roads, I arrive at a cozy family home marked by kids' bikes and toys in the front yard. As I ring the front doorbell, Shelly pops out and says, "You must be Cara. Come on in. Welcome to my home!" Shelly is thirty-seven years old, works part-time as a Certified Public Accountant, and is a mother of three children. Her son, Owen, is four and a half years old, the baby in the family, and is absolutely adored by his two older teenage sisters. As I step into the entryway and take off my shoes, I feel the love and warmth emanating from inside her home.

Elmo is on the television playing in the background, a dog is scurrying at my feet checking me (a stranger) out, and Shelly directs me to the kitchen. Shelly is incredibly warm and open and immediately makes me feel at home, as if we're old friends meeting for tea and a chat at her kitchen table. As I set up my recorder, she asks me, "Tea or coffee?" I reply, "Coffee." She says, "Absolutely, coffee, lots of coffee here!" Owen runs through the kitchen like a flash of lightning in a diaper and t-shirt, giving me a sideways glance and hurrying on his way. Shelly says, "That's my Owen, my baby." "Let me get him set up with his therapist and then I'm ready to go." I watch Shelly walk to the back porch and chat with Owen's occupational therapist, who comes to their home once a week to work on different gross and fine motor skills and sensory processing. While Owen jumps on the trampoline in the background, I ask Shelly to introduce herself and her family, and to tell me more about Owen. She states, "I've never found a definition for this, but he has very limited language. He can tell me if he wants juice or milk, but he can't say, "I played with so-and-so." He has some aggression problems, and he's not toilet trained. But he's very affectionate and playful, just not with children."

I follow up, asking, "If you were to describe Owen in just a few words, how do you describe him?" Shelly laughs and says, "Happy, sweet, moody," accompanied by a smile and an eyebrow raise. I then ask her to take me back to the very beginning of their family's experiences with autism. I am curious to learn the different interpretations of "the beginning," and all stories began in the same place. All mothers float me back to the precise doctor's visit in which they received the official autism diagnosis and how they felt in these first official moments. The diagnostic moment seemed to have a gravitational pull for all stories; it was the starting point for caregiver narratives and it's the starting point here for this book.

This chapter illuminates often forgotten aspects of caregiving, which reside in caregiver identity and that lead to the birth of the expert caregiver. Mothers here demonstrate how the current social experience of caring for autistic children can alter their own identities, social roles, and imagined family futures in a variety of ways. These internal identity ruptures are sparked by experiences of social exclusion and family marginalization due to entrenched cultural ideals of family and American family life.

The "traditional nuclear family," "domestic family ideal," and "Standard North American Family" are all sociological ways to capture the very precise notion of the American family that fundamentally excludes neurodiverse families and families with disabled members. According to Dorothy Smith (1993), the Standard North American Family is an ideological code defined in both terms of family structure—a heterosexual, legally married couple with healthy, able-bodied children—and in terms of family roles—a gendered division of labor within the family and home, in which women oversee the domestic labor, including all child and home care, and men work outside the home as primary breadwinners.

As an ideological code, this one conceptualization of the family operates as a universal norm through which all ideas of family, motherhood, and child-rearing are understood and constructed. In other words, this traditional notion of family is the reference point and center through which both individuals and institutions conceptualize and understand typical family roles and structure. Throughout these narratives, you'll hear how ideals of family are repeatedly referenced and reflect neurotypical norms and expectations—the ideal family is neurotypical according to our dominant cultural expectations.

Therefore, family is not simply a biological or physical entity, nor is it just a cultural performance. Family and family roles are also highly emotional and reside deeply in our subconscious, our self-identities, and visions for the future, which you hear in the words of mothers throughout this chapter. In their words, tangible changes associated with the autism caring journey—loss of homes and jobs, family tensions, and judgmental "bad mother" stares in public—can dismantle caregivers' previously stable identities and participation in dominant American family life. Although contemporary American families increasingly do not fit the traditional family model, this expectation is very much alive and well in the narratives heard throughout this chapter. The traditional nuclear family is very clearly the "home" in their ideas and scripts of family, motherhood, and childhood, which excludes neurodiversity and their social experiences as a neurodiverse family.

The entrenched neurotypical organization of society is a context to help illuminate the very personal identity changes that caregivers experience especially at the beginning of their autism caring journeys, which spark the desire to seek out alternative spaces and symbolic resources. Reoccurring experiences of shame and social exclusion serve as deep destabilizing hits to their own identities, which shapes the caring experience and prompts transformation at the level of identity.

By elucidating the depth of identity impacts associated with the autism social caring experience, this chapter provides foundational insight into explaining how and why so many caregivers work tirelessly to become experts and exceptional advocates for their children. Experiences with ableism, social exclusion, and tangible losses inform very personal struggles with identity, which form the starting point for transformation, and the birth of the expert caregiver. In becoming an expert caregiver, mothers actively reimagine their own identities and rewrite new, more inclusive family codes. Thus, this chapter functions as the first step in a larger story on how autism family caregivers become experts, and the complex and relational reasons for why they do.

"Since We Got the Diagnosis": The Primary Disruption in Family Narratives

"Since we got the diagnosis" is a phrase that I heard at the beginning of my conversations over and over again. The diagnostic moment seemed to have a gravitational pull for all stories; it was the starting point for the narratives of caring for autistic children. I met Catherine at a local coffee shop, where we sat outside for hours in the warm sun, and I listened to her tell me about her family and her experiences raising two autistic boys under the age of fifteen. After a description of her family and some basic demographic information, she began by saying, "Since we got the diagnosis, first one, then the other, our lives will never be the same." I probed, "What about your life has changed?" "Everything," she said: "Our daily routines changed. Where I planned to send them to school changed. My job changed. My husband and I are talking about possibly moving a few towns over because they have a better public-school system for children with disabilities. My whole idea of what our, my family's, future would look like completely changed. The diagnosis changed pretty much everything. It's a game-changer for sure!"

Catherine exemplifies what Arthur Frank (1995) refers to as "narrative wreckage," or the point at which the stories we tell ourselves about our families, our futures, and who we are lose coherence and meaning. The diagnosis prompts Catherine to question many of her deeply held assumptions about who she is and her scripts for her family's future. This moment is a profound disruption in all life stories, which first sparks a negative emotional response followed by a questioning or exploration process for most caregivers. Caregivers grieve not for the loss of their child, but for the loss of the nuclear family ideal and access to the master narrative of the Standard North American Family (Smith, 1993). Caregivers realize, for the first time, that their families may no longer match the Norman Rockwell paintings of ideal American families.

Like Catherine, the diagnostic moment provides a starting point for their stories but also represents a significant moment of realization that the "universal" dominant family form and the master script that accompanies it no longer fit their realities or their family's futures.

Everything that they thought was true and fixed, who they believed they were, and what their futures would look like started to become less certain, less fixed, and now blurrier. For example, Sarah, a caregiver of a six-year-old boy, stated, "I went to the appointment alone because I thought it was just a regular checkup. If I knew we were going to get an autism diagnosis, I would have at least asked my husband to come. So, I remember walking out of the doctor's, alone, in shock, and then driving home silently, still in shock. Once I got home, I put on a video for my son to watch and I went upstairs to my bedroom and cried for hours. I think I cried for days." I asked Sarah why she cried, and she replied, "For all of us. For what I thought his life would look like, for what I thought our life as a family would look like. For me, maybe never seeing him go off to college or walk down the aisle." She added, "I'm fully aware of the fact that my son may never leave the house. I love my son dearly and I'm so grateful for him and would not want him any other way, but I did have to go through a grieving process for quite a long time, before I was able to get to this point, to be able to talk about it." Here, Sarah shows how caregivers grieve for the loss of an idea of the American dream, embodied in the traditional American family—it's the romanticized *idea or image* she grieves, not the child.

More specifically, the official diagnosis prompts caregivers to reevaluate their own ideas of family, motherhood, and visions of the future—do everyday life scripts, routines, and interactions change? Do I need to send him or her to a different school? Can I hold the same assumptions and expectations for my child as I did before—that my child will go away for college, graduate, and land a great job, live on his or her own, marry, and raise a family? Lastly, what does it mean to be a parent of an autistic child? How does this affect me, my social roles, and place in the world? These questions and answers rely heavily on normative cultural scripts for traditional American middle-class parenting and family life, and they force caregivers to encounter their own uncomfortable ableist assumptions.

Most caregivers question if their children will be independent, will be able to secure a full-time job, or will get married and have a family of their own. Autism introduces greater uncertainties about their children's futures. These assumptions and expectations for their child's future are grounded heavily in heteronormative middle-class, white narratives. For example, Stephanie, a caregiver of two autistic boys, elucidates how these dominant assumptions and expectations for her sons have changed: "Daniel [Stephanie's husband] and I have talked about this. We don't expect our children to physically leave our house when they graduate. How some people expect their kids to go to a four-year college right after high school. I don't think that is going to happen. And it might be too early to say, but I just don't see that kind of stuff for our family." As seen in Stephanie's comment, the grieving process reflects a deviation from normative ideas of "doing family," which are, in this instance, especially class-specific. Previously held dominant middle-class narratives of American family life and pictures of the future begin to dissolve. The American dream of success—a married family with 2.5 kids living in a single-family home in the suburbs with a white picket fence and shaggy dog—starts to become unattainable, or crumble, for the first time for many of these families. Further, a part of this early process is the realization that this ideal family picture assumes ability and neurotypicality, which is largely inherent in the Norman Rockwell paintings and visual representations of the ideal family.

Mallory adds, "I know he's super smart, and I know he will be OK. And that's comforting because I know he will do something. It might not be something that I had envisioned for him, but he's smart and I know he's going to be independent, and I know he's going to be OK." Mallory's use of the word "envisioned" here is noteworthy, as it highlights the ways in which mothers' assumptions about the future for their children are shaken up. But she also worries about him, as most mothers do. She states, "I also worry all the time about him making friends. I'm worried about how people are going to perceive him and treat him. He's smart and he likes to talk about vacuums and whatever; I'm down with that. But other people are going to be like, what? And other kids already notice he's different that are his age, because he still wears diapers for one. It's like, his unwillingness to change is going to set him apart when he's older, I think." You can hear in her comments the beginnings of her exploration and acceptance of neurodiversity and what it means for her son, his future, and her own life.

In the following section, caregivers continue to share how the realities associated with daily carework challenge their social relationships, identities, and ability to "do family" normatively in a variety of social settings. However, in these stories of struggle, I hear the soft murmurs of change that transform caregivers' entire worldviews of motherhood and family and themselves.

"The Snowball Effect": Economic Disruptions in Family

We had our house, we were both working, and we had our baby. You know, awesome! And now, financially, with losing our house, our finances are terrible. Then, all of our credit cards were canceled; it's just been a huge snowball effect.

After retelling the diagnostic moment, mothers' narratives centered on describing a series of disruptive social experiences that destabilize both family and caregiver identity and their place in the world.

Specifically, caregivers described disruptions in three key domains—economic, marital and family relations, and public—that seem to increase in intensity and speed and to take on a life of their own, in a snowballing fashion. As Samantha sums up, "It's just been an out-of-control snowball since we got the diagnosis." The cumulative impact of persistent harmful snowballing disruptions affects mothers at their core, in which they no longer feel clear or confident about who they or where their family fits in the world.

First, economic disruptions were described as a result from the combination of expensive autism-related care and the frequency and extent of services that make formal, full-time employment outside the home difficult. Thirty-five out of the fifty women interviewed felt that geographic and housing changes were a result of expenses associated with healthcare interventions and support services, many of which are not covered or are covered only partially by insurance. Some have lost their homes or downsized. Others were forced to relocate to lower cost-of-living areas or to move in with family members. The socioeconomic changes that caregivers discuss result from structural problems in the American healthcare and social safety net, which does not provide sufficient and accessible resources to support complex and long-term child health needs.

Specifically, autistic children (and adults) can benefit from a variety of additional care services in the form of therapies, such as speech therapy, occupational therapy, physical therapy, and even equine therapy, that may or may not be covered by insurance or offered through the local public school district. Many families also seek out specialty programs or private schools that offer a more inclusive learning environment, which are both very expensive. Additionally, many mothers make the constrained choice to quit their jobs to be available for their child's care needs, which cuts their family earnings significantly.

Liz explains the financial strain that comes from the combination of high-cost interventions not covered by health insurance with the frequency of therapies and how she ended up quitting her job to care for her son:

My husband and I were both working at the time. Ok, so my son needs twenty hours a week in-home ABA therapy. How do we do this? So, I tried to work from home initially with him, and everything just went downhill career-wise. I couldn't return phone calls, I was trying to take him with me to property inspections, I got behind on my paperwork, and it was terrible. And I just put my hands up in the air and I was like, I can't do both, I can't do this, because when you work, you want to be the best at what you're doing. And people were counting on me. So, I threw up the white flag. I can't do it. I can't be there for you when you have a question about a house at whatever time and be there for my son too. So, I quit, which ultimately ended in us losing our home because we just couldn't make it on one income, which led to us living with parents for a year.

She finished by stating, "And my husband had to take a second job, so he's working two jobs and that's where we are now in a nutshell."

From an outsider's perspective, the large jumps in these stories leave out some information that could explain the shifting of events here. However, the ways caregivers choose to make these linkages among key moments in their story is telling. Liz's story exemplifies the feelings of powerlessness that many women felt early on as they described how they were forced to quit their jobs to meet their child's caretaking needs. With little to no negotiation, women took on the extended caring responsibilities. In a minority of cases, some mothers mentioned dividing caregiving tasks with their partners or negotiating work schedules to best meet their child's needs. But overwhelmingly, mothers simply took it on; the extra tasks were incorporated into everyday child caregiving, and in most cases, the husbands were on the periphery in daily carework and daily decision-making. As Kendra, a caregiver of two disabled children, describes,

My daughter has special needs too. She gets physical therapy, occupational therapy, and she has braces on her legs that she wears on her ankles—she has all that therapy too. It's hard for me to try to balance everything. And right now, my husband's in the city for work, and then he's going to come home for the weekend, and then he's going to be in Arizona all next week. So, it's really a mentally hard thing. I'm doing all this on my own. [She looks down and pauses.] I don't think he's met any of the therapists. He's not really involved in any of these aspects with the kids. [Shrugs.]

The absence of fathers' voices in this study speaks loudly to the gendered nature of carework. In this study, the unequal gendered distribution of carework is noticeably clear and aligns with the broader burden of care placed on women across the globe. Often, carework becomes a wedge that shifts the scales of balance overwhelmingly onto the lower-status party. In heterosexual families, this is women and mothers. Economic disruptions and an unequal care burden combine with additional familial strains that lead to uncomfortable feelings of shame that chip away at mothers' self-esteem and sense of self.

"It's Like We're in Two Completely Different Universes": Family and Relationship Strains

My husband went fishing a lot those first few months after we got the news. Our son is still our son; nothing changed—we know that. But, I think, for my husband, he needed some space to get his head around it. It was real in a way that it wasn't before.

Next, postdiagnosis economic challenges were linked with additional disruptions in the realm of family and marriage. For example, Stacey was particularly open in talking about the marital strains that emerged when her son was first diagnosed, largely due to different gendered coping mechanisms and opinions on parenting. She states, "It was a lot of ups and downs. I stayed up at night crying. My husband went to bed and insisted we not discuss it, so I sat in the other room with my books, and he did his thing." Looking back, she says, "There was a lot of fighting in that period.

When he's awake we're trying to pull it together, but suddenly we had these different ideas. I'm reading these books and think I'm now an expert. "We need to do this," I say. And he's parenting how he always has, because he doesn't get it or doesn't want to deal with it." She sums up: "Yeah, so it was a little rocky, for, I'd say six, seven months. Just different views, because at this point it's all our opinions. Nobody has a real idea of what we should be doing."

The pervasive uncertainties and ambiguities surrounding autism shines through here in Stacey's comment. "Nobody has a real idea of what we should be doing" is a powerful way to understand the impact of trying to care for your children in the best way possible, while receiving constant mixed messages from competing autism paradigms and professionals. Here, the contested autism landscape operates as an additional stressor in caregivers' lives that emerges in marital tensions. I gently inquired about their marriage today, to which Stacey replied, "We're great now. But there was that period where it was just, neither of us is going anywhere even if we're fighting because we have kids to take care of."

Tensions in marriages were mentioned as part of this "snowball effect" in ten interviews and primarily reflect highly gendered ways of dealing with stress and conflict. For example, Stacey's husband deals with the diagnostic news in a typically masculine way: he isolated himself and refused to talk about it or to share his thoughts and emotions. A level of emotional and physical disengagement is similarly shown by other fathers described as "gone fishing," "working more," and "not being available on weekends" for a memorable chunk of time following the diagnostic news. In all ten of these cases, the couples worked, or were continually working, through marital stressors.

Marital tensions are one form of familial stress that mothers discussed early in their journeys. However, more women discussed strains with friends and family members. Jessica describes this shift in social relationships: "We aren't around, like my coworkers, and even our friends with kids, we don't see them anymore. We have a new set of friends, the autism families, so those are the ones we hang out with." This shift in social relationships often occurs "just because it's easier." Easier how? I asked. She replied, "I used to try and explain when he was first diagnosed, what we were dealing with, because people were asking. But I don't think I could ever explain it right. I would just say, you know, that his brain is built differently, he has problems with speech, he has problem-solving issues, he has play issues. But what I would get was people saying, 'Oh, my kid had speech problems when he was younger.'" The dissolution of friendships results from a lack of understanding and explicit dismissal of one's realities.

Joanne echoes this theme of shifting social relationships due to dismissal and denial. She states, "My mom is still in denial to this day. She doesn't think he's autistic at all. She's read all the reports and everything. She just thinks everybody's overreacting." She continues to describe the ways her mother invalidates her son's disability: "She just thinks it's a behavior problem that I need to work on with him. She's like, 'Maybe he just needs a good spanking or something,' and I'm like, 'No. . . .' That's not the way I'm going to go here. She doesn't understand at all, which is a major problem because I now pretty much avoid my family, because we cannot even talk about anything. It's like we're in two completely different universes, and it's frustrating and useless."

"It's like we're in two completely different universes" captures the tensions in Joanne's family and shows the ways lack of understanding about autism translate to everyday family life. Because of false ideas about autistic behaviors, or unwillingness to accept autism, strains within immediate families often emerge regarding parenting. Family members give parenting advice to address a child's defiant or unruly behavior not knowing that the behavior is communicating distress, likely due to a sensory issue, as opposed to simply poor behavior. Neurotypical family members may not react to the loud screams at an amusement park, or the flashing bright lights at the movie theater, or scratchy clothing in the ways that the autistic child experiences them. When combined with additional neurotypical expectations for behavior (especially in public), the child becomes overwhelmed, flees, flails, or flops to the ground. Mothers learn to see these behaviors as indications that their child is distressed and needs help, while other family members label the child as naughty, defiant, or a spoiled brat who needs stronger discipline.

Marianne, a caregiver of a ten-year-old boy, has experienced a similar change in family dynamics. She no longer attends family holiday gatherings or sees her in-laws: "Last time we did Christmas was two years ago, and I explained ahead of time, he [her son] doesn't like crowds, he doesn't like to be touched, he does not want to be talked to. And even then, people kept going up to him and asking him, 'Oh, how are you, how are you?' and when he doesn't answer they ask again, and again, and again, until he freaks out. So, that was the last holiday with family that we've gone to. It's too stressful for everyone involved. We do Christmas by ourselves." Here, Marianne exemplifies many stories of close family members simply "not getting it," and, further, not being open to learning about autism or educating themselves about how best to support their grandchild or niece or nephew.

Additionally, it was not uncommon for many close family members to completely refute or resist the diagnosis, which reflects the negative social construction of autism. Early in these narratives, mothers commonly reported a lack of understanding about autism and how a child who appears visually and physically healthy can be disabled. Therein lies the crux of invisible disabilities: it appears very difficult for people to reconcile that a person can appear physically "normal" and even gifted while invisibly disabled by a society designed on neurotypical expectations. Further, it's not just the difficulty in making sense of these inconsistencies but also the explicit unwillingness to believe mothers and their children that fractures families.

Family strains and tensions emerge, because family members are unwilling to accept that the child is autistic, precisely because it has been socially painted as a negative, undesirable trait.

Mothers are the primary caregivers who have learned their child's triggers and how best to support their children. As Marianne described, she proactively spoke with her in-laws to make sure that everyone could have a positive Christmas experience.

She states, "I explained ahead of time, he [her son] doesn't like crowds, he doesn't like to be touched, he does not want to be talked to." Asking a lot of rapid-fire questions places a large demand on a child that can quickly trigger a fight-or-flight reaction, which is what happens with Marianne's son. So many mothers share stories of feeling unheard—"They don't believe me"—or dismissed—"They think I'm overreacting." These reoccurring experiences of dismissal or shame by loved ones hit mothers hard, particularly when combined with additional negative social experiences in public.

"Some Days It's Hard to Take. It's Not Ever Easy Being Judged": Disruptions in Public and Bad Mother Stares

I think my little guy works really hard to do what comes natural to other kids. I think that there's people that give dirty looks to people in stores and you don't know the story, you don't know why the kid's doing that. Don't give dirty looks, you know. And don't judge people. You don't know what they're going through. You don't know what their kid's been through.

The feelings of isolation or being othered increase with a variety of negative social interactions and experiences of public shaming in everyday life. For example, Terri's experience with trick-or-treating on Halloween exemplifies how common autistic behaviors can disrupt participation in public everyday life with negative consequences:

> Halloween is my favorite holiday ever and all my other kids, you know, my step-kid and my daughter loved it. So, I got a Halloween costume for Max, Superman; he knew it, and we went out trick-or-treating. And two minutes into it, he went up to the door, but he wouldn't say, "Trick or treat." The lady kept saying it to him over and over, and he just had a complete meltdown. It took my husband and I both to carry him back to the car while he screamed, and everybody was, "Oh my god," because he was

beating on us. And Christmas was coming, so I just found myself thinking, "I can't do Santa. I can't do anything. We might as well just skip the whole holiday thing."

In this case, Terri's previously assumed and taken-for-granted participation in cultural rituals and traditions, like trick-or-treating on Halloween, is challenged, which increases her feelings of exclusion from dominant American family life.

This trick-or-treating example demonstrates the cultural expectation that young children are verbal, can easily engage in a scripted interaction with strangers, and enjoy doing so. When they do not, the inclination is to push for conformity and compliance, for the child to perform according to the cultural rules regarding Halloween, and when they fail to do so, blame is individualized and placed on the child and parent. These are examples of the subtle ways that neurotypical standards are deeply entrenched in everyday family social life and American cultural traditions.

Similarly, Anne, a caregiver of a five-year-old child, exemplifies the anxieties that many caregivers feel when participating in daily mundane activities in public spaces: "I'll never forget the many trips to the grocery store, to Walmart, to the mall, when he would start screaming at the top of his lungs in the carriage. God, if you could have seen the stares and looks of disgust I've received from so many people! It was as if I was torturing my child or something." She continues, explaining the reasons for her son's behavior: "Come to find out, he is overly sensitive to lights and sounds, so he gets overstimulated very easily by things we do not even hear or see at all. Like, he would be fine until we got to the freezer aisle in Safeway. I now realize the freezer section has a ton of low-grade buzzing, and the lights go on and off as you walk through. I learned to leave the freezer section to the very last part of my grocery shopping, then I literally run to the check-out, and try to get out of there as fast as possible, to avoid all the nasty looks."

Like Anne, most neurotypical people would not notice or be affected by low-grade sounds or blinking lights that are present in every trip to the grocery store. However, for children with sensory processing sensitivities or difficulties, stimuli like fluorescent lights, strong smells, and background noises in busy, crowded spaces can cause overstimulation and physiological distress. What happens when any child is overstimulated and distressed? And what if that child is nonverbal and cannot explain why the child is distressed or what the child needs? From the outside, it often looks like bad behavior and overly permissive mothers who cannot control their unruly child. Based on these neurotypical assumptions, mothers are often shamed and sanctioned with "nasty looks" or "bad mother stares" in public settings.

Many mothers described uncomfortable and unsettling experiences in public spaces, in which they received "looks of disgust" and "bad mother stares" by strangers, as a result of their child's misbehavior in public. Anne poignantly explains how many caregivers internalize the negative attention they receive throughout their daily carework activities, which functions as a threat to their identity "After experiencing so many instances like this, I developed a bit of a complex and some irrational fear of going out in public. I mean, when people look at you with such disgust, and I'm literally running out of stores as fast as I can, it's hard not to! I've learned to work around it, and I care less now. I've moved on. But, it's unbelievable how judgmental and *not* understanding people can be. Other parents for that matter—they should know better!" (She shakes her head, disgusted).

"Some days it's hard to take. It's not ever easy being judged," says Katie. She continues, "Sometimes it's like I have a real 'F it' approach. And sometimes I feel like I have to explain his behavior to everybody around us. And so, I haven't really navigated through how to deal with it. And I don't take him to Walmart or the grocery store. I go when he's in preschool. And I think that people who had two kids would do the same thing, so it's kind of not really autism, it's just taking any three-year-old."

As illustrated in the quotes above, the snowballing series of economic strains, changes in housing or jobs, tensions in marriages and familial relationships, and judgmental interactions in public lead caregivers to question, "Who am I?" Empirical experiences of profound change and social marginalization function as a challenge to one's self-identity—who they thought they were, and would be, and what the future of their family looks like.

Frequently, caregivers stated verbatim, "I feel like I lost myself." For example, Carole describes her transformation from an ambitious, outgoing career woman to a stay-at-home mom: "I gave-up my career, I went to school, and I have my bachelor's. I'm a really social person, always working. I always thought I would be a working mom. Now look at me, rarely leaving the house. I never considered that I would be a stay-at-home mom."

Here, we can see how external social realities associated with autism carework disorient caregivers' previously stable sense of self-identity. Furthermore, these stories of grappling with new family identities are grounded in traditional middle-class discourses on American family life. Here, Mary demonstrates this process:

> I had this idea of what my life would be like. "Oh, we'll have kids, and we'll go camping and we'll go boating, you know we'll have fun and do all these family things." But, when your kid has a different view, or needs so much more care, and won't do any of these things—. For two years he wouldn't stay anyplace else besides his own bed, so that shuts out camping, or going away on vacation, or anywhere for that matter. This has been hard on me and my husband; we've had to totally transform our ideas of what we thought family life would be. I would be lying if I didn't say that because of all of this, I've been diagnosed with depression and an anxiety disorder and I'm on medication for both, which is something that I have never, ever dealt with in my life.

As this quote indicates, identity ruptures and psychological stress reflect one's displacement away from the normative center, and from access to previously held group memberships and imagined family futures. Here, the idea of going away on family vacations, engaging in fun leisure activities, like camping and boating, are important parts of Mary's identity as a mother and wife accustomed to a certain middle-class lifestyle—these are perceived to be expected, "normal" parts of middle-class family life. Her exclusion from these activities is an assault on who she is as a mother, wife, and woman.

The disruptive and tumultuous experiences at the beginning of their caregiving act as the catalysts for transformation—transforming ideas of self and family, and of autism. These early experiences force mothers to encounter their own internalized ableism and to sit with it. The new awakening to the fact that societal norms are set up in a way that disadvantages their child and family is a motivating factor for change in themselves, for their worldview, and for seeking out different social spaces and more inclusive communities. Their feelings and experiences are valid to them and reflect the broader uncertainties that surround autism, the lack of public understanding and acceptance of neurodiversity, and the institutional obstacles that intensify feelings of marginalization as a neurodiverse family.

It is through daily carework and family activities that caregivers experience subtle and not-so-subtle deviations from the ideals of contemporary middle-class family life. For Carole, it was losing her job and becoming a full-time stay-at-home mother; for Liz, it was being forced to quit her job and the loss of her home. For others, it is everyday conversations with family members that demonstrate a complete lack of understanding of their child and situation; it is husbands spending more and more time at work, and it is judgmental glares and stares received in public spaces when a child is "behaving inappropriately." It is the compounding nature of these small, micro-level disruptions and changes that elicit a disruption, too, in caregivers' identities and performances of family. This negative reinforcement from family and societal interactions prompts caregivers to begin questioning what a family is and how it operates. In turn, these dynamics challenge their assumptions about hegemonic white, middle-class narratives of motherhood, gender, and family life and reflect upon their newly emerging place in the world.

"It's the Little Things": Reframing Family Codes and Caregiver Identity

We laugh about things. Gary's first question was, "Where's my balls?" And, you know, it was real, but we cracked up, because you have to. I don't want depressing. I know what it's like, so I don't need to read that other people are having a hard time. I want to read their laughter.

In response to the dynamic relational process between self and society, caregivers use their social roles and carework practices to move through feelings of exclusion and uncertainty and to repair ruptures in self-identity. The previous stories of snowballing disruptions that were told with such urgency and anxiety in each breath seemed to slow down, and a levity took over in caregivers' voices. They shared intimate family moments and talked about their children with reverence. As Maria articulates powerfully here, "It's the little things":

> We have those moments where Billy isn't in the middle of some kind of tantrum, and he will do something or say something, and the things that make everything easier for us are when he does something that we look at each other across the room and smile, because we're both thinking the same thing. It's our nighttime routine, where we're lying on either side of him in bed for twenty minutes, and he's cuddling or singing—all those little things that he can do, we notice. And we notice them together—the girls [her daughters] notice some, my husband and I notice some, and it just makes us feel more like a regular family. "Oh look, he just did . . ." So, it's the little things.

Seemingly small moments of pride and contentment become major events in some families' life stories and serve as significant forces in the rewriting of new ideological codes for family. Attention shifts to center the moments of deep connection with her husband and children.

The ways in which these heartwarming events are told are central moments in the shift away from narrative emphasis on struggle and loss to new feelings of pride, hope, and inclusion. Maria continues to describe moments in her day and family life in a loving and appreciative manner: "Well, he loves snuggling, getting under the covers. You know, he's really into kissing right now [laughter]. Hard love—he smashes his face against your cheek." You can hear the warmth in Maria's voice as she recalls snuggling at night with her son and engaging with him, as a family, in the things that he loves to do—swinging, jumping, and going on walks. She says, "Things like sitting and doing puzzles or blocks is not something he really enjoys doing. He wants to be running or swinging or jumping. So, we go for a lot of walks. He loves that, you know, with Dan and me." Caregivers also beamed with pride telling me about their child's special interests, accolades, and academic strengths. As Maya states, "Everybody has things they are good at. And Zack is very bright. When he was in kindergarten, he knew all the states and capitals and he was reading at four years old."

In the telling of these heartwarming family moments, you hear mothers' perspectives changing. The way they see and understand themselves, their child, and their family changes. The centrality of structural disruptions and snowballing losses are replaced with sweet family moments and a sense of calm. In this narrative change, caregivers seem less stuck in the heaviness of the past and more content and grounded in the present—enjoying the little things and not taking the good days for granted. Meanwhile, mothers' own relationships with themselves and how they understand their role as primary caregiver also change. This narrative turn is similar to anthropologist Gail Landsman's (1998, 2008) research with mothers of disabled children, in which she found a similar duality in mothers' narratives. She summarizes, "Most mothers I interviewed tell what at first appear to be two stories, one in which they hurt for their children and for their own losses and another in which their experience of mothering a disabled child has taught them that their children are, after all, normal and their own lives enriched" (p. 92). Accordingly, reoccurring patterns in the data highlight the persistent structural context specific to disability and "normality," which informs the perceptions and experiences of caring for disabled children.

A part of this narrative transformation process includes caregivers' thinking differently about their role as caregiver and the responsibilities and potentials it involves. Emma, a caregiver of a five-year-old boy, described how reframing her role allowed a greater sense of personal empowerment and agency to decision-make: "Sometimes, I resent it. That I have to do all of these extra things for him, alone. Sometimes I don't agree with what is recommended for him. Besides my other autism mom, I can't talk about this with anyone else. No one understands all of it. So, it's a burden, but it's mine. And that makes me feel powerful. That's how I see it. He needs me right now and I can do this; this is what I do now!" Anna echoes this juxtaposition of the burden of care with agentic decision-making and the value of experiential knowledge: "It's taxing to make huge life-or-death decisions on your own, but at the same time, I don't have to compromise, and I can go with my gut. I can do what I feel is right for my child and I don't have to listen to anyone else. I know what is best for my son."

When asked about sharing the decision-making in particular, Colleen states, "My husband's opinion is always 'What do we think?' He'll go with whatever I think, which makes things easier, I guess. We don't have to fight about it, you know? But it's hard to deal with when the decisions feel like life or death." Mary adds, "I feel like if anyone knows what's best for him it's me, and I feel pretty confident in that because nobody spends as much time with him as I do. Nobody knows his quirky things, his ins-and-outs, what he'll eat, his therapists, better than I do." She continues to state, "I've had to not lean on my husband or anything for support because you really can't—I can bounce some stuff off of him and get his ideas but ultimately, like what we do is going to be up to me." I asked for an example, and she said, "Right now, I'm deciding if he should do a couple of different programs, and I kind of bounced it off my husband, and he kind of shrugged his shoulders and I'm like whatever, I'll figure it out."

Many women here describe frustrations with their husbands sharing the decision-making load in particular that is a part of everyday family and household management. Accordingly, here we see how the heteronormative strict gendered division of labor persists in many of these families and arguably is exacerbated due to the extensive carework activities and responsibilities taken on by mothers. In this way, expert caregiving functions as a means to uphold traditional notions of family and familial roles. At the same time, expert caregiving also chips away at hierarchical family relations by providing sources and spaces for women to gain power and combat feelings of exclusion, as well as challenge ableist assumptions about what a family looks like.

Specifically, mothers' frustrations are ultimately reframed overwhelmingly as a space to assert their agency, which is underscored in the confident way in which they speak about being the expert on their children. Over time, many caregivers come to realize how they are the single most important and vital resource involved in the care of their child, and this fact plays a large role in rebuilding ruptured self-identities and empowering caregivers and families. As caregivers gain self-confidence through skills and experiences learned via expert caregiving, they also subvert the highly unequal power dynamics inherent in the gendered division of labor.

Further, it is through their everyday carework that these mothers are encountering new ways to see themselves and discovering new, hopeful, and deeply satisfying futures for their families. It is in the everyday decision-making, doctors' visits, therapy appointments, teacher follow-ups, and conversations on neighborhood playgrounds that mothers are understanding themselves, their families and their role in them, and meanings of autism anew. Individually, they are shifting their own perspectives on motherhood, family, and autism through their everyday carework, and in turn, chipping away at the hegemony of the traditional nuclear family. In this way, carework holds intense emancipatory power to facilitate change in very tangible, pragmatic ways.

Writing New Family Codes: The Vital Role of Symbolic Resources

The calm and content family moments shared by caregivers above are important ways to balance the overwhelming negative series of "snowball effects" described above, and more broadly, in the literature. As Sara Green (2007) notes, the literature disproportionately focuses on the negative emotional impact on caregivers caring for children with invisible disabilities and disorders, which are often presented in false binary ways—good/bad or negative/positive. I intend for my study to blur this binary representation by showing the nuanced realities associated with families living and caring for children with invisible disabilities.

Autism family and caregiver resource groups and in-group public spaces provide a refuge from the daily experiences of "otherness" with which these families live. Specifically, all interviewees participated in at least one of the following: caregiver resource or support group, play-date group with autistic children, or meet-up family/ social group. The opportunity to meet other caregivers and families, who share similar stressors at family holiday gatherings, struggles with their child's teachers, or the latest snide comment they received while grocery shopping, is validating and significantly mitigates feelings of social exclusion and isolation. Participation in these mediums also provides caregivers opportunities for knowledge and skill-building that assist in the redefinition of self and family.

Liz emphasizes the vital role support groups have played in her life:

> The first time I attended a parent and caregiver group, I think my life changed. Until then, I never met another person with an autistic child, and I found myself asking so many questions and just going up to everyone afterwards asking about their children and their experiences. I went home and I felt less out-of-control about the whole thing. I felt like I now know people who I could

turn to when I need to make decisions, find a new school tutor, or doctor, and who will listen to me and actually understand what I'm going through. My family and friends listen, but they really do not get my life or my child or what I'm going through, so they can only do so much.

Liz feels limited in the degree to which she can connect with her family and friends, since they don't understand her experiences. Therefore, she turns to her local parent support group for pragmatic information, support, and understanding, which helps her to feel more in control as a caregiver.

All caregivers described the positive functions of support or resource groups to provide a sense of belonging and answers to real, domain-specific questions, such as recommendations for local neurodivergent-friendly dentists, after-school programs, or the best therapists. Some caregivers pushed their engagement further by organizing special social groups and outings specifically for children who are typically excluded from these activities. For example, Aimee started a local autism family social group because "I think everyone likes to feel a part of something, where you feel understood, and like you don't have to be constantly explaining yourself. More specifically, she states, "I was thinking that it would be nice if we could go do things, like go to gymnastics, and not have to worry that people won't understand us. So, I called, and they said, 'Yeah! Bring the group in.' And that's just kind of how it started. A place to go do things where, if there's a problem, I'm not embarrassed. You want to explain, but there's 150 people out there, you can't go up to everyone and say, 'He's hitting me because there's something wrong, not because he's a brat and I'm a terrible mother.'" She continues to give a recent example of how symbolic resources allow caregivers and families to just be themselves, without any judgment, even for just a few hours, surrounded by people who simply "get it": "The last time we were at gymnastics, my son took off his clothes in the two minutes that I was talking to another parent. But, it wasn't humiliating. I just got his clothes, chased after him while we all laughed. It's nice to have that. People get it."

Consequently, these support networks and community groups help caregivers to push through the previously described spectrum of identity confusion and "narrative wreckage" (Frank, 1995), by creating new meanings for the autism caring experience and new ways of being for caregivers. For example, Lisa describes the vital function that community support groups and networks play in redefining her orientation to autism and her son: "By attending every group and resource meeting that I can around here, I've really learned how to think differently about autism, and about my son. But now, I've learned not just therapies but also to look at autism and my son's behaviors differently—that they're not all negative, bad things, or detrimental to his life. Like, because of autism he is amazingly observant and so smart. He is so smart, it's crazy! I really credit these groups to helping me to shift how I think about my son and my own role taking care of him. It's changed our relationship for the better." Here, Lisa underscores how symbolic resources can present ways to reimagine oneself and one's children and family. Through active participation in local support group meetings, community events, and social groups, previous snowballing disruptions are replaced with gains in social roles, self-identity and purpose, and new ideological codes for the American family.

Social interactions with friends, families, and the lay public shape the different narratives of caring for autistic children, while participation within meso-level autism community groups plays a pivotal role in transforming self-identities and conceptions of family. These narratives highlight the fact that both identity and the family are neither a static thing nor a predetermined entity, and they are contingent upon social interaction. Inclusion in the autism community affords caregivers the ability to reflect differently on their experiences and to change their perspective particularly on deviance and normality.

Rupture-Repair Cycles and the Birth of the Expert Caregiver

This chapter began by describing stories of narrative disruption from caregivers' perspectives, which highlight the power of dominant neurotypical cultural norms and ideals about motherhood, family, and ability. Here, family challenges—financial stressors, housing changes, marriage and relationship strains, and public shaming—are told in a snowballing and relational fashion as if autism is the driving force. However, these challenges and strains result not from autism or their child, but from the social construction of autism and disability as deviant and the social processes of ableism that structure our daily lives. The ways in which these events are plotted and perceived especially in the early stages of diagnosis reflect the biomedical construction of autism as deficient in an ableist society.

Importantly, how mothers make sense of the diagnosis and their early experiences of social exclusion and isolation are the roots that spark transformation in caregivers' own sense of self that lead them to engage in extensive sets of practices and roles that push the bounds of family carework and good mothering. The process by which the caregivers' sense of self is disrupted is a critical, yet underplayed, part in understanding why people become expert caregivers in the first place. Therefore, the purpose of this chapter is to detail the birth of the expert caregiver, and specifically to center caregiver identity and the deep internal transformations that occur in direct relationship to broader cultural norms on motherhood, family, and autism as key pieces to understanding the broader phenomenon of intensified carework.

What exactly distinguishes expert caregiving from traditional caregiving? What types of labor do expert caregivers do, and why? And how can everyday carework by lay mothers hold the power to transcend hierarchical boundaries between lay and professional while also shining a light on entrenched cultural assumptions about disability? Chapter 3 begins to address these questions by detailing the different mechanisms through which caregivers maximize their education and skills as a variety of lay/experts, and in doing so, push hierarchical power dynamics and subvert false boundaries of multiple worlds.

3
Making Sense of Difference
Building the Expert Caregiver Toolkit

Some public libraries have these cozy private rooms with couches that make you want to curl up and escape into a book for hours. I reserved one of these spaces and arranged to meet Danielle there one evening. I found the room, sat down at the table, and waited for Danielle to arrive. A few moments later, a young woman with long blonde hair, casually dressed and coffee in hand, came bustling into the room. "So sorry; mom time is always ten minutes late," she said. "No worries at all; you are right on time," I replied. "Gosh, look at me. Can you tell I don't get out much?" We both have a little laugh, and then Danielle settles in, and she introduces me to her family.

Danielle is thirty-one years old and has been married for over twelve years to her high school sweetheart. She is the mother of one son, Lucas, whom she described as "funny, quirky, and loving." Lucas was diagnosed as autistic at three and a half years old by a child psychologist through an independent autism evaluation. I asked her how she understands and explains autism to other people, and she said, "That's really hard for me to answer actually, because when typically you think of autism, you think of little or no eye contact, repetitive motions, they're kind of lost in their own world—that's not my son at all. I still struggle with that," she continues, "because if I say oh it's a social deficit, or he might have specific mannerisms that are kind of strange, stuff like that, people just look at me funny." She adds, "I know how he's different, but I don't really know how to express that, really. Even after all these years."

To try to understand better how Danielle makes sense of difference and autism, I asked a few follow-up questions. She responded by explaining her first concerns were with Lucas's speech: "I was trying to get him speech therapy since he was one. When he turned two, he only had maybe five words." I asked if she brought this up with her doctor or anyone else, and she said, "I told his doctor, and she was like, 'You know, give him some time, wait 'til he's two and a half, and then go from there.'"

"So, two and a half comes along, we go to the doctors, and I asked again, 'What about the speech therapy? What do we do about that?'" Danielle said that she prepared for the visit by keeping notes on her phone, a "speech diary," as she called it, in which she would note the words and sounds he said each day and even took some videos. "He said a handful of words that you teach babies—'up,' 'water,' 'eat,' you know? Only single words, and I mainly noticed it when we went to the park and saw other kids his age talking up a storm." I asked her what prompted keeping the speech diary, and she said, "I knew to be prepared this time. Come on, he's two and a half years old and barely speaks. Don't you think this is at least worth a referral or investigating a bit more?" she said. "It's not really my style, but I got a little pushy with the doctor. I'm not the wait-and-see type anyways. Plus, with all the waitlists around here, I just don't want to waste any more time."

We talked nonstop in this little room, where I felt like I was talking with an old friend catching up on life. We heard a voice come over the loudspeaker that said, "Library is closing in thirty minutes." Danielle said, "Wow, I can't believe I've been chatting away for two hours. Geez, I guess I have a lot to say!" "I have a babysitter for another hour. We can continue if you want," she added. I replied, "Of course, that would be wonderful." We made our way outside to a table in front of the library and sat down, and Danielle picked up where she left off, at times teary-eyed. We chatted into the night, until she had to leave to relieve her babysitter. As I waved goodbye to her in the empty parking lot in the dark, I realized that a lot of mothers are seeking a listening ear, for someone to hear and believe their stories, and give them the space to talk about it. To have someone, even a stranger, believe what they are saying and validate their experiences is significant, because many mothers struggle to be heard and taken seriously when they notice differences with their child's development. I met Danielle early on in my research, and our almost-four-hour-long conversation, partially in the dark, in front of the public library has stuck with me ever since.

Beginning with the simple notice of difference in the child's behavior, this chapter describes the process through which autism carework intensifies and expands to take on a variety of professional roles and skill sets. Specifically, the jurisdiction of unpaid carework expands past traditional carework boundaries to include all of the following: (1) scientific observation and analysis; (2) diagnostic tracking of behaviors, triggers, and changes and diet or supplement therapeutic protocol design; (3) proficiency in comprehending and appropriating medical literature and knowledge, navigating bureaucratic health care systems, securing resources through professional agencies, coordinating across agencies, and child advocacy; and (4) teaching (homeschooling), lesson planning, and specialized knowledge and modalities specific to PT, OT, and speech therapy.

Through the processes of taking on a variety of professional healthcare roles, caregivers learn entirely new skills, bodies of knowledge, and ways of interacting and communicating, which allow them to overcome structural obstacles in the caring experience. First, caregivers become lay diagnosticians to make sense of inconsistencies and developmental differences, and to navigate the winding road to a formal diagnosis. Then, they become a variety of healthcare professionals to gain access to evaluations and services and to maximize the quality of life for their children. Everyday carework expands far beyond the lay private sphere into professional formal spheres of medicine and health care. Caregivers engage with medical diagnostics, scientific research and literature, and various support therapies, with what feels like life-and-death consequences. As a result, sophisticated expert caregivers emerge who are highly educated on autism, able to employ medical jargon and specialized discussions with professionals, navigate institutional bureaucracies, and act as multiple therapists, all while advocating for their children and caring for their families.

The demonstrated inability of medical professionals and formal healthcare infrastructure to address the wide-ranging uncertainties and needs involved in the autism caring experience is paramount to understanding why parents go to the extreme lengths that they do to educate and train themselves to help their children and why and how they turn to a diverse set of allies to do so. In this chapter, I build this concept of the "expert caregiver" by first demonstrating the major institutional limits and challenges involved in receiving an official diagnosis and being taken seriously in medical interactions. Next, I show how caregivers maximize their health literacy and take on a variety of different professional roles, extending traditional notions of carework.

An Introduction to Neurodivergence: Becoming a Lay Diagnostician

You know, you've got a panel of six professionals who just tested your kid, but they can't tell you what's really going on.

For most families, the road to an official autism diagnosis includes many twists and turns, bumps, and dead ends. Only eight out of fifty children (16 percent) in this sample received an official diagnosis before the age of three, although they had presented atypical traits since infancy. The remaining forty-two families embarked on a journey to the autism diagnosis, which lasted anywhere from six months to five years. These cases provide valuable insight into the roadblocks involved in receiving a diagnosis, which sparks extensive health carework, and how and where lay families gain greater institutional access and control.

Most mothers knew something was different about their children from infancy. You'll hear more from these mothers who noticed developmentally atypical behavior and their experiences in a fragmented healthcare system later in this chapter. However, I want to begin with a few interesting cases in which autism, or any significant developmental issues, were not on mothers' radar at all and came as a surprise. These cases show the messy line between typical and atypical child behavior and development, and why it is so difficult to receive an official autism diagnosis in a timely fashion. For example, for Aimee, "It was his daycare actually who insisted that something wasn't quite right." She proceeded to walk me through her potential concerns and how she rationalized them: "I thought his behaviors—up to two he was pretty typical, and then he just kind of quit playing with toys, and I thought, 'Eh, he's just weird,' you know? He was lining them up instead of playing with them. But, it didn't ring a bell." She continued, "Huge temper tantrums, but I figured he's just spoiled; I mean he's a little one and the girls spoil him rotten. So, I thought, 'He's just kind of a brat.' The aggression—then he started banging his head on things, and that's when his daycare said, 'I can't keep him if you don't get him tested.' So, I called our pediatrician immediately."

"What happened next?" I asked. She continued, "I called his pediatrician and said, 'My daycare says I have to get him tested for something; she doesn't know what's wrong.' And he sent me the M-CHAT [Modified Checklist for Autism in Toddlers-Revised (M-CHAT-R)] and I sent it back and he said, 'Well, from this I should be referring you, but you were just here a month ago and everything was okay.' And it was, sort of."

I inquired further about the inconsistencies found here, and she replied, "Yeah, that's the thing, it's super confusing. You can check 'no' on some things, but they're all deceiving.... Yes, he did have the thirty-five required words, but I guess I didn't think about the fact that I hadn't heard them in weeks. So, I just checked 'yes'—he knows thirty-five words.... And nothing prompted the pediatrician to be concerned either. He's a good guy; I like him." Eventually, based on the M-CHAT autism screening results, Aimee's pediatrician referred her to the local hospital's autism clinic, where they conducted many tests and confirmed, "Yep. He has autism."

Aimee's narrative of the road to the diagnosis is puzzling, and yet common, in many instances. Many mothers discussed how their children were screened regularly for autism, always passed, and later were diagnosed as autistic. Although her son was completely nonverbal at three years old and displayed aggressive and repetitive behaviors, it was not her pediatrician or any other medical professional who alerted Aimee that her son's behaviors are atypical. Instead, it was the daycare worker's insistence that "something was just not right" that served as the mobilizing force in Aimee's taking action to understand her son's differences.

Dana, a mother of a now-five-year-old boy, described her son's complicated road to the diagnosis as a battle: "I would describe this process, mainly at the beginning, as a battle. I felt like I was constantly fighting for something—an appointment, to get off a waitlist, for a referral to someone, to get into a research study, for my family to understand, for my boss to let me cut back to part-time and keep my job. A battle, I tell ya!" "But we found our way, and we got there and it's a lot less rocky now; we have a system," she continued.

The first "battle" for many mothers was discerning "typical" versus "atypical" behavior and having someone, anyone, believe them. As Rebecca states, "Looking back, there were red flags, but he's our only child. I was an only child. So, we didn't spend a lot of time taking care of younger children or whatever. We didn't have an idea of what is typical or normal." "But he would do the arm flapping. I took him to the beach, and he wanted to just stick his hands in the sand over and over and just kind of, you know, feel it? Just noticing the waves, the ocean, digging with a bucket, and flapping," she said. "That's when a little tick went off in my brain like, 'Hmm that's a little weird, right?'" She then describes concerns with her son's speech, and the realization that he was not retaining words: "He was really slow to talk, and we weren't particularly concerned because we had both been slow to talk. He could say his alphabet; he could count to twenty at eighteen months. He would count over and over. Like he'd go up and down the stairs and count: one, two, three. He lost all of that, but at the time it was ok because he would pick up new words." However, she then recalled the moment when her son "wasn't retaining the words." She said, "We would hear them, you know, for a day or two and then not again. I got obsessive about keeping track of new words, how often he said them, and when he stopped saying them."

I asked what happened next: "What did you do with this information?" "Well, my mom and mother-in-law were a little concerned and suggested taking him to a speech therapist. So, we did that." Rebecca then tells me that the speech therapist noticed some sensory seeking behaviors and suggested that she "look into sensory processing disorder" and "getting a neuropsychologist evaluation." "So, we went to that, and then it's like oh, yeah, you know, he has autism," she said.

Whether they knew from the beginning that "something was different" about their child or they were caught off guard by an autism diagnosis, a common theme in mothers' stories was uncertainty and needing to make sense of puzzling inconsistencies. Most mothers responded to growing uncertainties and frustrating interactions in the clinic by becoming a lay diagnostician. A lay diagnostician is a non–medical expert or scientific professional who actively observes, tracks, diagnoses, and treats a group of traits, behaviors, or symptoms as a medical condition, or in the case of autism, as a neurotype and disability.

Caregivers take on the role of lay diagnostician by carefully and closely observing, noting, and analyzing their child's behavior: In what contexts do their behaviors change (i.e., when and where do meltdowns most often occur)? Does he have repetitive behaviors? When do they seem to intensify? How does she play? What does she do around other children? How many single words or phrases does he have? Can he jump on two feet and one? Can he hold a pencil correctly? Does she keep up physically on the playground with peers? Does he retain words? Is she losing vocabulary? Does he look people in the eye? On playgrounds, at playdates, gymnastics, soccer, and swimming classes and in public spaces, mothers now start paying careful attention to their child's behavior in comparison to others of the same age, and they track triggers for upset and meltdowns. Then, the data compiled from these observations are presented to the appropriate medical professional.

"I noticed that . . ." "Is it normal to . . ." "Should I be concerned about that . . ." and "At this age . . ." were all phrases that mothers repeated to their pediatricians to broach a conversation about difference and potential concerns about developmental delays. For example, Rachel described the response by her pediatrician to her concern that her son was acting "differently from her older daughter at this age" and not talking at the age of two: "I told him my concerns and he said, 'Well, he's not talking yet but that's within the range of normal.' We just kind of went through the regular checkup and shots and nothing came up. So that's when we sought out a speech therapist on our own for the nonverbal and communication issues."

Like several other mothers, Rachel interprets her son's atypical behaviors as a medical problem—primarily as a speech and language issue—which she then treated in its matching biomedical form, through speech therapy. Rachel's interpretation of her son's speech delay and her resultant action to seek professional speech and language support make sense, since the biomedical model is the dominant paradigm for understanding difference. Autism is not on many mothers' radars when they first start seeking help on their own. Similarly, Brynn, a mother of a two-year-old autistic child, describes similar experiences of dismissal by her pediatrician, which leads her to independently diagnose her child's behavior challenges and gross motor delays and to seek out experts in these two areas accordingly. She described to me how "the concerns we had—I don't think she [the pediatrician] understood them." Consequently, they switched doctors "after a few years." I asked her to tell me more about what motivated the switch, and she said, "It was a lot of the things, the valid concerns that we had with our son. It was just—she brushed them off as 'He's strong minded and strong willed.' No! I know my son can be strong willed and I know he can be stubborn, but there's something else here."

What do you mean by "something else here?" I asked. She replied, "Besides behavior stuff, I was really concerned with some other things. Like, I noticed he would use one side of his body more, and looking back he was late in everything—to roll over, to crawl, to walk—everything." She continued, "I know these are typical gross motor delays, so I found an OT [occupational therapist] person to help with this, and I called a child psychologist to try to figure out the behavior problems—or just some advice or something, you know? He recommended ABA. I did this completely outside of our doctor's recommendations."

Like Brynn, most mothers knew in their gut that something was different about their child, though they struggled to put their finger on what exactly was different, and medically there were no clinically significant red flags. Invisible disabilities have more perplexing qualities, in which children are developmentally typical or advanced in many ways, although they struggle in other ways, and physically may appear able-bodied or "normal." The diverse ways that autism presents itself coupled with public misunderstanding exacerbates the complexities involved with diagnosing autism and making sense of autistic behaviors. Simply put, children may slip through the cracks more easily, and it appears to become a caregiver's job to make sure they do not.

Consequently, caregivers are tasked with meaning-making, discerning if there are concerns with their child's development in the first place, and then compiling evidence to present to an authoritative body for formal help. As part of their daily carework, they track their child's behavior, research typical development milestones, research and contact local providers, attempt to enroll their child in several evaluations for services, educate themselves and family members on autism, and continue to work their way through winding bureaucratic processes.

In the narratives above, caregivers play the role of a lay diagnostician, which includes a learned skill set of data collection, evaluating, interpreting, and tracking behaviors and triggers, as well as analysis. Then, they present their concerns to the pediatrician, who typically recommends a "wait-and-see" approach. In most cases, mothers are not satisfied with the passive response, and they seek out specialists or aid elsewhere. When pediatricians do not refer them to speech or occupational therapy, they do it on their own, privately. Private therapies and autism evaluations are typically more expensive than services acquired through a referral. Therefore, the ability to push back on pediatricians' "wait-and-see" response necessitates the financial means (and time) to do so. It's important to note that many mothers and families do not have the luxury of money and time to push back, which often extends the road to the diagnosis, and most importantly, the services that the diagnosis grants (coverage by health insurance or eligibility and funding by public schools).

Accordingly, this section provides further depth in conceptualizing the lay diagnostician as a key mechanism to make sense of the child's behavior and to combat institutional obstacles and the dissatisfaction felt within clinical interactions and the formal healthcare system. You may be asking, but why is a diagnosis important? Especially if autism is best understood as a form of disability, neurotype, and identity? If the biomedical model's emphasis on disease or disorder is flawed and damaging, why seek out a formal medical diagnosis? For the mothers in this study, and many others who experience diagnostic uncertainty, an official diagnosis serves the following key purposes: (1) official diagnostic labels are a prerequisite for testing and a variety of services and accommodations, which are vital to support autistic children and provide a better quality of life, and (2) official diagnoses function as a significant form of validation for children and their primary caregivers. Without a diagnosis, many children cannot even qualify for programs or services, and insurance will likely not cover healthcare costs. The official diagnosis is the gatekeeper for insurance coverage and access to services in health care, education, and other publicly funded programs. Therefore, mothers' carework intensifies to overcome the bumps and dead ends on the road to an official diagnosis, because the stakes are so high.

All children in this study had received an official autism diagnosis, and once the diagnosis was granted, mothers' daily carework pivoted away from diagnostician tasks to health literacy. After the diagnosis, mothers no longer need to be lay diagnosticians, but instead become incredibly literate medical consumers who blur the lines of lay and professional to secure integral services for their children. As a result, a sophisticated expert caregiver emerges who is highly educated on autism, able to engage in medical jargon and discussions with professionals, and able to navigate institutional bureaucracies, all while caring for their child.

Expert Caregiving Tools: Education, Skill-Building, and Lay Expertise

Educating myself was my priority at the very beginning. I threw myself into reading everything, listening to every podcast I could find, spending days on Google searching and searching and emailing every contact I could get my hands on. My family always knew where to find me—sitting at the computer!

To combat the many uncertainties and frustrations involved in the autism caring experience, parents seek out information and resources in every way possible. Throughout this process, they become an expert caregiver, and the ultimate medical consumer, while simultaneously blurring lay/expert boundaries. In this section, I detail the rationale and motivation that drive these practices, the actual form, mechanisms, and spaces in which they occur, and the resulting proficiency in comprehending and appropriating medical literature and knowledge, navigating bureaucratic health care systems, securing resources through diverse professional agencies, and experimenting with self-designed interventions.

One of the most prominent themes in the process of becoming an expert caregiver takes the form of health literacy. Health literacy is defined by the Institute of Medicine (2004) as "the degree to which individuals have the capacity to obtain, process, and understand basic health information and services needed to make appropriate health decisions." Health literacy requires a complex group of reading, listening, analytical, and decision-making skills, and the ability to apply these skills to different situations. For example, it includes the ability to understand instructions on prescription drug bottles, medical education brochures, and doctors' directions and consent forms and the ability to negotiate complex health care systems (Institute of Medicine, 2004). The mothers in my sample all engage in diverse health literacy practices and integrate them into their carework, though to different degrees. Some caregivers exhibit exceptional levels of health literacy, while others employ more passive strategies or struggle with the limits of lay/expert boundaries.

For example, Susan, a part-time administrative assistant with an associate's degree in computer science, exemplifies a remarkably high level of health literacy that extends beyond traditional carework to include exceptional information-seeking, gathering, and analysis skills: "I read everything! Medical clinical books, research studies, parent blogs. I put my kid in every study I can, I talk to the doctors, I seek out new people. . . . I go to every talk and lecture and event I can. I ask questions; I don't hold back. I've seen just about every specialist and autism-related doctor in the state! I ask other parents for advice. I just try to gather as much information as I can and keep on it. Studies are coming out so fast, so I have to keep on top of the latest reports." Like Susan, many caregivers funnel their time and energy into becoming experts on autism itself, spending hours each day reading clinical books, research studies, textbooks, and online blogs; conducting extensive web searches; and contacting support groups, service agencies, and professional experts throughout the world. These expert parents are incredibly well informed, self-educated, and connected. Liz represents this practice of maximizing her health literacy, in the interest of the well-being of her son: "I spent forever on Google, just researching by myself. You just keep looking. I mean I had books on the verbal behavior approach, and pivotal response therapy, and I have every book there is, reading them and trying to figure out, 'Would any of this really work?'" Liz is referring to different models and approaches in behavioral therapy, of which there are many.

During a stressful and exhausting time, information and connection provided a sense of structure and control, a way to minimize anxiety and uncertainty, and a way to maximize individual sense of agency and decision-making capacity for caregivers. As Lisa summarizes, "If I can just read everything, I can make the right decisions, I can make informed decisions, and I can help my son. . . . Because that's all we are trying to do here, make the best decisions for our kids. No one else is going to do it, and no one will give you the perfect answer!" The lack of a "perfect answer" or explanation, I think, drives a lot of the extreme health literacy practices that mothers describe.

The majority of mothers feel very alone and unsure in terms of what is in their child's best interest. So they read and watch and listen to everything with the illusion that if they just know everything there is about autism, then they are doing their job. Generally, the search is targeted toward better understanding and resources to minimize harmful behaviors or treatable health issues (like GI upset) and increase independence and quality of life. As Beth says here, "I don't want my son to change. I would like him to be able to maybe learn things like social cues, so that he doesn't say offensive things to people, or make friends more easily, stuff like that. I don't want him to change who he is. I would not change him for the world; I'd just like the world to open up to him." The "world opening up" to children like Beth's son is key to understanding the dominant neurotypical context that frames caregivers practices.

I get the sense that the stakes are incredibly high here—that mothers feel that if they miss something (the latest research, best therapy model, school accommodation, etc.), then they have let down their child and have failed as mothers. This rationale that drives mothers' intensive health carework practices is an important part of the story.

Further, these actions now become necessary parts of mothers' everyday carework. In addition to traditional domestic labor, including cooking, cleaning, childcare, and eldercare, mothers now are lay diagnosticians and health-literate researchers who compile, read, and analyze and engage with diverse literatures. These are highly specialized skills that many of us spend years (ahem, decades) in school learning, and these women take it on because they feel they have to—it is what they need to do to care for their children—and no one else is stepping up. Again, the lack of institutional support here is apparent.

The fact that mothers spent their few moments of quiet at the end of every night after the kids are asleep annotating journal articles, emailing researchers, and trying to find local specialists that practice play-based speech therapy reveals the flaws in care structures that leave massive holes in understanding and support. In the wee hours of the night, in between laundry cycles or finishing up work for their paid jobs, mothers are submitting packets of intake forms for new occupational or speech therapy or searching for local equine therapy programs that may take insurance. This is unpaid and generally unacknowledged labor. Additionally, the information seems stuck at the individual level—in other words, each mother is telling me about very similar experiences, literacy practices, and researching the same questions or local therapists, and each one is doing it alone.

The majority of women in this study have at least one other child, are married, and take care of a home and family, and many work at least part-time outside the home. To become an exceptionally literate expert caregiver requires enormous amounts of time, energy, and financial resources. The books, expensive supplements, membership fees, and tangible resources all are costly, and not everyone can or wishes to engage to the same intensity or degree. Each caregiver employs different health literacy strategies to address that caregiver's unique social locations and needs. However, what everyone lacks and is searching for are professional advice and answers to various questions that remain unaddressed or impossible to answer.

What I find here, is that most clinical studies and texts and the latest scientific findings and premier research studies do not address or begin to tackle the questions and areas of need that autism caregivers are seeking: how does this information directly relate to my everyday life? Therefore, it is easier to understand why the autism caring experience requires extensive parent-led self-education, research and experimentation, and the confidence to ask questions, to discern information, and to act on earned knowledge, all alongside, but not (always) fully within, the formal institution of medicine and health care.

The Appropriation of Expert Knowledge and Playing Professional Roles

A major dynamic in becoming the expert caregiver and applying one's health literacy involves the appropriation of expert knowledge. To circumvent and push back against professional or formal limits, caregivers practice the appropriation of expert knowledge as a means of minimizing the distance between expert and nonexpert and gaining entrée into previously off-limits realms. The appropriation of expert knowledge can serve the following purposes for lay caregivers: (1) to understand and engage with research and literature (i.e., in case studies, research studies, and reading paperwork), (2) to gain legitimacy in the clinic and to engage in more democratic dialogue in doctor-patient interactions, or (3) to gain access to different support services, with the goal of minimizing treatable medical symptoms (i.e., sleep disturbances and GI issues that significantly affect everyday life) and improve quality of life. In my interviews, I hear lay women appropriating expert knowledge, citing research studies and statistics, and using clinical language and jargon to describe and communicate their experiences and interactions. Lay mothers become experts of different kinds, which is particularly salient in the realms of contested and complex medical disorders and disabilities.

This process by which lay caregivers embody expert roles and scripts can be understood as engagement in "lay epidemiology" (Davidson, Smith, & Frankel 1991), "popular epidemiology" (Brown, 1992), or "street science" (Corburn, 2005); a lay way of knowing that is based in part on an appropriation of expert knowledge by nonexperts. All these concepts are simply different ways to capture the same fundamental goal, which is a pushback, even in the smallest ways, against top-down knowledge and hierarchical practices in health care and medicine, which do not adequately reflect caregivers' experiences. When the experts are unable to provide the answers or the assistance that parents need, parents themselves become the experts, and a primary means to do so is through the adoption of expert knowledge and learned proficiency in medicalese. To date, these concepts have yet to be connected to carework.

Medicalese refers to the use of formal medical terminology and semantic qualifiers, or the ability to read, understand, and use medical jargon appropriately. For example, to explain what autism is, Allie cites almost verbatim its technical biomedical characterization, and one can see the appropriation of clinical language in her response: "I constantly find myself explaining what autism is to other people. I've created these little scripts, you know, that I've pretty much memorized, based on what I've read. To other adults, I say my son has a complex neurodevelopmental disorder, which includes repetitive behaviors, and communication and social impairments. But to kids, like in his school or on the playground, I usually say, 'Jimmy has a different brain and he understands and processes things differently.'"

Similarly, throughout our interview, Sarah incorporates the latest statistics and research findings into her family's general autism narrative. For example, when describing the rationale behind her remarkable health literacy skills, she states, "So, why do I do all of this research to educate myself, call experts, and browbeat my way into the top doctors' offices? Most of the specialists have like a six-month waiting list, you know. One doctor that I wanted to see, it was going to be over a year to see him." She continues, "I do it because I notice people take me more seriously now, when I can show that I read the research and know the words and can talk like them. I can call, 'Bullshit,' when I know they are not telling me the right thing or completely brushing me off. Like I know the therapy options out there, I know the statistics on what has worked and hasn't, so don't lie to me."

Sarah calls it like it is—she's tired of being dismissed, delayed, and passed over, so she studies the research, learns the language, cites statistics, and uses the right words to be taken seriously in medical encounters. Many caregivers assert scientific knowledge in their interactions as a means to gain leverage with professionals and formal organizations, not just in health care but also when dealing with teachers, case workers, and school boards. In other words, the learned use of medicalese is a strategic way to blur lay/expert boundaries and to gain power in hierarchical institutional spaces, in which lay caregivers traditionally occupy the subordinate position.

An additional mechanism that challenges lay/expert boundaries and professional domains lies in the practice of caregiver-led research and experimentation with diet and supplement therapeutic regimes. For example, Charlotte believes strongly in the role of supplements and diet to address some of her son's challenging behaviors and health issues, like regular constipation and stomach upset, which are common in autistic children. She told me that she heard from a friend about a local naturopathic doctor who was giving lectures in town on alternative autism therapies: "I thought, I mean, really, what do we have to lose? Nothing! Except that it's pretty expensive." The doctor advised keeping a food diary to track possible food allergies.

Consequently, Charlotte "started by keeping a diary of everything" her son ate and drank "and noting any triggers or flare-ups to try to assess allergies or what could be making things better or worse." She did this for a while, and then started a supplement protocol. She states, "Following the protocol, I started introducing one supplement—vitamins and stuff—at a time, noting any changes. And then another and another. When things got worse, I took him off it. I also noticed dairy and gluten did seem to aggravate symptoms sometimes, which is typical with these kids, so I took him off dairy, but gluten is too difficult for a picky eater. So, I'm still experimenting with this and changing doses and keeping my diary. These changes have definitely helped with his sleeping problems. I also notice less tantrums; he seems calmer."

Like Charlotte, many others discussed experimenting with nonprescription homeopathic supplements and over-the-counter vitamins to treat many of the common health issues associated with autism, such as anxiety, depression, sleeping problems, gastrointestinal issues, and food allergies. Most caregivers learn of these treatment forms through self-researched books, web-based searches, and autism-community listservs and referrals, not from formal literature or professional recommendations. For example, Debbie discusses how she experiments with diet and supplement changes with little professional oversight or direction, hoping to minimize some of her son's physical aggression and hyperactivity: "My son can be really aggressive, so I've been looking into how to decrease the aggressive behaviors. I read a lot about a vitamin called L-carnosine for calming. So, I bought it off Amazon. And the company I bought it from is called, like, 'Autism Coach,' so it's for autistic children. But it's a liquid form that I put in his chocolate milk every morning. And I think that he's gotten less aggressive and it helps with digestion and stomach problems. I know that there's a lot of autistic kids [who] have problems with constipation and stuff, so I'd recommend it . . . but it's fifty dollars a bottle."

All these books and in-home diet and supplementation regimes are not covered by insurance; they are expensive and require large amounts of time and energy from caregivers, with little guidance. Jennifer provides a critical perspective by honestly addressing the difficulty to maintain and keep up some of these caregiver-led alternative therapies, with sometimes few results:

> We tried the GFCF [Gluten Free Casein Free] diet because everyone was saying we should. I noticed no changes, but it was so hard to do, so I quit doing it. We kept him off milk because I noticed diaper rashes went away, and I'm lactose intolerant, so I thought, "OK." So, he drinks almond milk—that's all we kept. There's also been periods where people have said, "Oh, these supplements." And I've bought them, and tried them, and noticed no change. I don't think that I believe all of that works,

I just usually keep my opinions to myself when people are talking about it. . . . You're desperate enough to try it, and if there's any improvement in that period, then you're a believer.

Here, we see how many caregivers act as nutritionists or dieticians who research available diets and supplements, create their own protocols for their children, track effects, and then tweak the protocol as they see fit. Several scientific skills are being learned in the process of research, protocol design, data collection, and analysis, as mothers take on the role of nutritionist to help their children.

Mothers learned additional skills associated with the formal realms of speech therapy, physical therapy, occupational therapy, and ABA therapy—the primary therapies recommended to help autistic children. It is common for autistic children to have delays with speech, language, and verbal communication. With a referral, speech therapy can be covered by insurance; however, it may be limited in frequency. Children may need therapy two to three times a week in order to see improvements, though health insurance or the public school system may only cover one session a week. Therefore, caregivers are tasked with learning and leading therapy sessions at home. Many caregivers talked about their therapy "homework" and the many activities that they have been told to lead and replicate at home. For example, Samantha walked me through a typical after-school routine, in which she squeezes in "therapy homework" each evening: "So, I pick up Austen from daycare around 5 P.M. I start dinner and find the weekly notes from his therapist—the things we are supposed to practice. Depending on his mood, I try to do some OT activities combined with speech stuff. So, we can hit on both."

While the water for pasta comes to a boil, then, Samantha is leading an exercise to work on Austen's fine motor skills, while also integrating some speech therapy work. "Other days, we'll do some PT exercises, and I try to work on speech stuff too. I make sure to pull up the PT exercise sheets so I'm doing it right, and sometimes we watch YouTube videos if I'm not sure. Speech stuff is easier because it's really just me talking to try to get him talking more," she continued. She then details how she usually leaves Austen to finish up so that she can finish dinner and get everyone to the table to eat. "We eat dinner. I turn on the TV for Austen, and then I help my oldest with his homework."

I asked her how she felt about the therapy homework and after-school routine, to which she replied, "Eh, honestly, it's a lot. Things are very hectic. Sometimes I think to myself, 'What the heck am I doing?' I'm not a speech therapist; I didn't go to school for this. I went to business school; this is way out of my league. But, they tell me I'm doing it all okay." Samantha's after-school routine that squeezes in caregiver-led therapies with typical family domestic labor was very common. Many other mothers described feeling stressed just anticipating the after-school events. They are stressed because of the time crunch after school and before bedtime, in which they are trying to meet multiple demands, while playing multiple different roles, some of which they do not feel totally comfortable with or capable of doing. Many mothers described feeling unsure when asked to take on sprawling professional skills, for which they were never formally trained.

Mary astutely says, "So many times in the middle of working with my daughter, I say to myself, 'How the hell did I become an occupational therapist?' I never even heard of occupational therapy before it was recommended to us. But, damn, I'm pretty good at it. Imagine if I went to school for it!" She laughs. Many mothers did not just follow the homework given to them by their child's therapists but also went further to research activities and watch YouTube clips for more ideas. Here, they are learning and practicing general skills in research, lesson planning, and teaching, as well as specialized knowledge and modalities specific to an array of autism therapeutic supports.

Others transferred formal training that they'd received for their own careers into caretaking tasks now required for their children. For example, Alexandra is a mother of three children under ten years old, and her youngest, Will, is four years old and autistic. Will receives OT, PT, and speech therapy twice a week. Luckily, she was able to find and afford a local private center that offers all three services, so she can combine all three therapy sessions into one trip. First, she describes to me the mental gymnastics that she does to coordinate the schedules and logistics for all three children. "My two oldest are in school all day, so that's when I take Will to therapies, doctors' visits, et cetera. He goes to part-time preschool, so we have time. After school, I shuffle my oldests to soccer and ballet. Will usually tags along, and then dinner." Then, there's the family "homework time": "'We all have our homework,' I like to say. My oldests have actual schoolwork to do. My husband supervises them. I work with Will on whatever we're supposed to be doing for his therapies." She continues, "Luckily, I was a teacher. I went to school to be an elementary school teacher so this is right up my alley. It's all teaching, you know—the therapies—I follow the handouts from his therapists. The work is really in how to motivate him and how to keep him on task. So, these are totally things I know how to do."

Additionally, because of extensive bullying experiences in K–12 schools, some parents choose, or are forced, to homeschool their child. In my sample, only two mothers chose to pull their sons out of public school to homeschool them in a safe environment more conducive to learning. Both children were experiencing extreme levels of anxiety due to bullying and social exclusion at school, which led to behavioral issues in the classroom. They were not learning or academically performing because school was "terrifying" for them. For example, Lizzy describes what led her to remove her child from second grade in her local public schools: "He would throw huge fits every morning because he hated school so much, not because he doesn't like learning or can't learn—that's not it at all; he is incredibly bright. It was because of all the social stuff—other kids constantly picking on him, calling him names, not sitting with him, teachers interacting with him as if he was stupid. You know how vicious kids can be to anyone different!"

Further, both mothers feel that they made the right decision for their children, as reflected here by Lizzy: "We had no plans to homeschool my kid. Luckily, when I was in college I worked in some after-school programs, so I guess I feel comfortable teaching.

It just got so bad that there was no other option but to pull him out. So, he's doing really well with the homeschooling, and I know it was the right decision." Lizzy exemplifies how the autism caring experience can extend the caregiver role far beyond the realms of health care and childcare to include formal classroom teaching.

Interestingly, mothers rarely discussed outsourcing any of the carework. There were mentions of babysitters to help with transporting kids to and from school and after-school activities, eating a lot of takeout to alleviate cooking, or "the house is a mess all the time," but I believe that these mothers are doing all of this very much on their own. Not once did I hear a mother talk about her husband being the primary at-home therapist—the one who researches, plans and organizes, and leads the therapy work—or the main contact for communication with therapist or teachers. Some husbands engaged in this work by taking children to appointments, "helping out" or "supervising" home lessons when the mother was unavailable, but it was mainly described as within the mother's realm of responsibility. Therefore, the unequal gendered division of labor in families discussed in chapter 2 expands here as caregivers take on more roles and responsibilities. In doing so, boundaries between expert and lay and public and private are blurred.

The Expert Caregiver Toolkit: Blurring Lay/Expert and Private-Public Boundaries

I hate the idea of not doing something that could have helped. So, I Google and I read and I spend too much time thinking about it. And probably he's got just what he needs—I don't know. And I harass people all the time: "What do you think of this?"

Throughout this chapter, we've seen how becoming an expert caregiver involves the blurring of different lay/expert boundaries. Mothers demonstrate how they repeatedly take on and off multiple hats, playing the role of mother, driving kids to soccer practice, making dinner, giving hugs and asking their kids about their days, and then function as professional therapists, school and health advocates, and case managers. The diverse professional roles and responsibilities that these mothers perform every day, combined with traditional childcare and household labor, explode the category of carework and role of caregiver. The boundaries between the domestic sphere and the formal professional sphere are also blurred. Mothers are acting as diverse professionals (unpaid), completing formal specialized tasks, within the private sphere of the household. Further, they are doing so alongside, or even during, the completion of traditional family carework.

Mothers are researching fine motor skills activities on their phones while cooking dinner and watching TedTalks on autism while folding laundry. They are modeling speech with one child, while checking another's schoolwork. They are answering emails for their paid job, while reviewing an Individual Education Plan (IEP) draft and making notes for the upcoming meeting and thinking about what to make for lunch tomorrow. It's a lot—mentally and physically. It's a lot for even the most privileged caregiver who has access to the time and financial means to meet these conflicting and extensive demands.

The stakes are high, and the lack of support from professionals drives mothers to seek out external resources or become the professional themselves, thereby pushing formal boundaries. A conversation with Aimee best demonstrates this complicated position in which caregivers sit between lay caregiver and medical expert, and especially illuminates the decision-making process that mothers engage in: "With the therapies, you're always second guessing. A couple weeks ago I was thinking, 'Maybe MAPS [the Medical Academy of Pediatric Special Needs program] isn't a great idea; he's been hitting more.' And I'm thinking, 'Okay, I haven't seen any really big improvements in the last few months; maybe it's time to call it quits.' But I don't know if that's the right choice, so I'm afraid to make it."

"So, what do you do then?" I asked. She replied, "Well, I asked his teacher and his therapist, and I got opinions from fifty people to tell me whether or not this program is good for my kid. It's frustrating, because you just want someone to tell you the right answer, or if this will help. Somebody tell me what will help, and I'll do it. But it always comes back to me."

"Always comes back to me" signals that mothers are given loads of recommendations and referrals—Read this! Try this! See Dr. X!—that represent widely different orientations to autism, only some of which are evidence based, and individuals are left to reconcile conflicting information and decision-make even when they do not feel confident doing so. Australian sociologist Kylie Valentine's (2010) research with parents of autistic children found similar tensions surrounding health literacy and decision-making in autism health carework. She states, "Whatever the explicit expectation placed on them, parents of newly diagnosed children are inevitably placed into this enormously dense, contested field of information and interpretation" (p. 956).

By noting caregivers' frustrations with vast uncertainties and structural flaws particularly at the beginning of their diagnostic journeys, we are better able to understand why parents throw themselves into intensive health literacy practices. Health literacy practices provide the tools necessary to be informed caregivers who are taken seriously in formal, traditionally masculine spheres and can complete the expansive carework required of them to maximize their child's well-being.

However, it is important to note the significant limits and constraints involved in becoming an expert caregiver, maximizing one's health literacy, and playing the role of numerous experts. First, even the most advanced and sophisticated collective of resources will not always be able to provide the knowledge necessary to guide the next steps on the autism journey. The ultimate expert caregiver is still a layperson, not a credentialed professional.

Expert caregivers are limited in different ways by their social location, cultural capital, degree of institutional access and formal ties, lack of professional credentials, and official membership in the formal institution of medicine. An expert caregiver is not a medical professional; the patient-physician role is clearly defined; yet the findings in this study show differing ways in which the lay-professional boundaries are simultaneously complicated and blurred.

Second, the ability to access, develop, and expand the expert caregiver toolkit relies on having the financial means and class-specific competencies to do so. More specifically, the ability to push back against professional dismissal, research and secure diverse support therapies, navigate bureaucratic healthcare systems, and challenge health insurance denials are all expensive in terms of money, time, and mental bandwidth. Further, these normative parts of autism carework also require confidence, perseverance, social connections, knowledge, and communication skills necessary to engage in extensive institutional negotiations with authority figures. In other words, becoming an expert caregiver necessitates both financial assets (economic capital) and social assets (social and cultural capital) and therefore can reproduce class inequalities.

Sociologist Pierre Bourdieu (1979) delineated between these three types of capital which are relevant to understanding differential experiences with expert caregiving, or why some people may have an easier or harder time becoming an expert, securing services, and advocating for their child. "Social capital" refers to social networks and relationships that can produce valuable resources, and "cultural capital" refers to the knowledge and skills, such as language and education, that are advantageous within institutional realms; both forms of capital are integral to becoming an expert caregiver and inform differential experiences therein.

Caregivers in positions of higher social standing, particularly of higher social classes, have access to the economic, social, and cultural forms of capital that those of lower socioeconomic status do not. Specifically, social connections can produce referrals to top physicians, help to get a child off of a waitlist, or enable access to support programs that were previously unknown. Cultural capital—"knowledge about 'the rules of the game'" (Lareau, 2015)—affords the language, knowledge, qualifications, and skills necessary to become a health-literate, confident, and capable advocate that blurs lay/expert boundaries. Class privilege affords caregivers the cultural knowledge to advance in dominant institutions and to overcome institutional sticking points in autism journeys.

Further, in discussing the ways parental social class informs educational experiences, Annette Lareau (2015) states, "In particular institutional moments, cultural knowledge is crucial. And in some instances, cultural training is not learned on-the-job as an adult, but appears to be linked to lessons in childhood" (p. 22). Therefore, it is important to underscore the value of class-specific cultural knowledge as crucial in the ability to become an expert caregiver, which is largely intangible and invisible. And, further, to remember that children are watching all of these experiences detailed by their caregivers in this chapter—how they experience successes and failures, and how other people, especially in positions of authority, react and respond to them. In these interactions, children are learning very clear lessons about how the world works and their place in it, and differential advantages are transmitted along class lines that significantly impact their future life trajectories.

The stories in this chapter begin rooted firmly within each family's isolated home and private doctor-patient interactions. Here, many parents observe atypical behaviors in their children, which are dismissed or minimized by their pediatricians during well-child visits. Then, parents turn away from the medical institution and look elsewhere for information or answers that the formal healthcare system fails to provide. Through the process of embodying the roles of various healthcare professionals, a sophisticated set of health literacy skills is developed, and families begin to overcome diverse institutional obstacles in health-seeking and access to care. These diverse roles and skills become integral parts of their toolkit and describe distinctions associated with expert caregiving. The autism expert caregiver is well read and current on autism scientific literature, tracks their child's behaviors and triggers, appropriates medical language, designs diet and supplement protocols, and is skilled in multiple therapeutic modalities.

All these characteristics and tasks extend the typical idea and responsibilities associated with traditional carework. Additionally, it is important to see these information-seeking and skill-building practices as realms that allow caregivers small yet significant moments that allow them to assert their agency in a seemingly powerless experience. Through gaining access to clinical studies and literature, by Googling everything and anything on autism, attending professional lectures, and asking questions of anyone who may listen, caregivers are not just increasing their knowledge of autism or their child; they are becoming experts in shaping their experiences to achieve the best care and support for their child. Information gathering and skill-building are powerful; they allow caregivers to guide and create their experiences with medical professionals and healthcare institutions, peers and family members, and with autism itself. In doing so, these practices shed light on the importance of amassing combinations of social and cultural capital (knowledge, skills, networks, and resources) to allow caregivers to feel capable of providing the best care possible for their loved ones.

Medical diseases and disorders that follow a more linear trajectory, which are diagnosable with a blood test or scan and have a clear prognosis, treatment regimen, and stable institutionalized body of services, involve a different caring experience. In normative biomedical illness experience, there are less ambiguity and uncertainty—you know whom to contact, where to go, what to do, what therapies to try, what specialists to see. Institutional policies and procedures exist to help patients receive aid. The roadmap for how to meet a patient's needs and how to care for the patient is relatively linear, defined, and straightforward, and it simply exists.

However, for families with disabled children or children with medically complex chronic health issues, oftentimes every step in the journey is full of questions and takes place within a highly fragmented system, in which professionals do not speak to each other and support services are disconnected from one another. We see how many mothers start by seeking out independent services—speech therapy to address speech delays, OT for gross motor delays and sensory sensitivities, PT for physical challenges, and ABA for behavioral issues—all unlinked from each other and from autism. Therefore, the building of the expert caregiver toolkit illuminates the lack of infrastructure to make sense of and support developmental differences, which includes access to appropriate diagnostic bodies and affordable services.

So in place of timely systematic procedures, access to professionals, and coordinated care, mothers take it all on through their carework. In this chapter, caregiving takes place largely within each family's personal home and family. Imagine fifty mothers separately in their own homes each day reading, researching, and acting as diagnosticians and therapists with their own children. Here, carework is largely conceptualized as an individualistic endeavor and performed within the bounds of the micro-level private, intimate, domestic sphere. Chapter 4 extends the jurisdiction of carework beyond the walls of the home and into the local community and public institutions, which is the next step on the journey to become expert caregivers.

4
Transcending the Private Sphere
Extending Carework into the Community

On a warm sunny evening in June, I walk up to the front door of a beautiful home, reach to ring the doorbell, and am interrupted by a young boy's face peeking out from behind the door. He opens the door more fully and says, "Hello," before I can press the bell. I hear a voice in the background yell, "Zachary, what did I tell you about opening the door for strangers!" I feel guilty, knowing it was my fault that this sweet little boy is getting in trouble. Fiona rushes out, a bubbly, petite, brown-haired woman in her thirties, and says, "You must be Cara. Come on in!" She puts her hands up and says, "I'm in the middle of making dinner and my hands are dirty; otherwise, I would shake your hand! If you don't mind me cooking as we chat, please take a seat." I take my seat at the kitchen table crowded with school papers, drawings, and mail while Fiona proceeds to cut up vegetables.

She says, "Sorry about the door situation. We've had some issues with Zachary opening the front door to strangers, so it's something we are working on." I reply "I see; no problem at all," and ask her to begin by telling me more about Zachary and her family. She jumps right in: "Well, we're a family of four. Brady is our oldest; he's twelve. And Zachary just turned eight on Sunday, and he's our youngest. Brady was diagnosed with ADHD in third grade and that's what we thought was going on. Then Zachary came along, and it was in preschool when we started noticing something was going on. We didn't know what it was." She continues to walk me through the early concerns she noticed with Zachary: "He wasn't playing with anybody. He was just different. He was doing the same things that our older son was doing"—and later, she noticed "serious issues" in first grade.

Her children's diagnosis story is interesting. Since her older son was enrolled in an ADHD clinical study at a local hospital that was seeking siblings, she enrolled Zachary. One of the clinicians said to her, "I think you need to have both of the children reevaluated." So she did, and Brady was diagnosed autistic and ADHD, and Zachary autistic. I asked her to tell me more about the "serious issues" she mentioned with Zachary in first grade, to which she replied, "He did not even complete first grade. We pulled him out of school. It was like the last two weeks because the teacher was just ridiculous. He was in the principal's office every single day." He was sent to the principal's office every day due to behavioral issues that Fiona described as related to the teacher's lack of understanding of autism: "He was having daily massive, screaming meltdowns, and the teacher wouldn't have any idea what to do. That's not my son." She finishes by stating, "Clearly, his meltdowns are communicating something is very wrong in the classroom and no one was doing anything about it, except sending my kid to the principal's office and then calling me to come get him. So, I pulled him out."

Over time, Fiona was able to discern more about what was happening that was triggering Zachary at school. She learned that his favorite things were being used as rewards and punishments and taken away from him when he didn't comply: "He's always been allowed to bring this little stuffy and a green frog eraser to school, and he holds them, and it gives him comfort. Well, I learned that they were being taken away as punishment. Well, he broke. You know, no one told me this. I had to find out in bits and pieces from my son." She continued, "Frankly, I was pissed. I called to meet with the principal and told him that my kid needs a one-on-one aide at school with him for next year." Fiona proceeds to tell me extensive ways in which she has advocated for both her boys in the school system, for one-on-one aides, autism training for all faculty, and transferring them out of certain classrooms due to bullying. She engages in intensive carework in her children's elementary school, with teachers, administrators, and even the school board. She fought for and won programmatic changes in her local school.

Fiona fights hard for resources and changes in school to help her children, as well as their young neurodivergent peers. Her immediate goal is to minimize the suffering and challenges that her own children experience in school, mainly by securing them resources (i.e., in-class aides) or removing them from harmful situations. However, she is also very much concerned about "all the other kids who do not have a mom like me" to advocate for them. As she begins to tell me more about her project to get mandatory autism training for all teachers at her sons' schools, Brady appears hungry for dinner: "Mommy? Excuse me." Fiona replies, "Yes? Did you finish your homework? Did your brother finish his homework?" "Yup," says Brady. "Wonderful. Let's eat!" Fiona says. Everyone settles in at the kitchen table for dinner.

So far, we have seen the exceptional lengths caregivers will go to receive an official diagnosis and vital support services for their child. In doing so, carework is a personal, micro-level endeavor that predominantly takes place within the intimate, private sphere—within the home, family, and individual healthcare interactions—and is self-focused and wholly oriented toward meeting the needs of the caregivers' own individual children. Therefore, the beginning steps in the dynamic process of becoming an expert caregiver are largely disconnected from one's surrounding community and meso-level forces. However, once caregivers feel that they are informed and capable of meeting their own child's daily needs, their caregiving becomes less myopic and isolated, and instead starts to broaden in scope to include the local community. Once caregivers feel confident in their ability to care for their own child, many express a desire, and in some cases a responsibility, to help other families on their autism journeys. They are no longer just laboring on behalf of their own child; they now work *for* others and *with* other families to secure resources and knowledge and build more inclusive communities.

This chapter demonstrates the ways in which expert caregiving is marked by the extension of caring labor outside one's private home and family and into the surrounding local community. Here, expert caregiving becomes a public, prosocial practice, through which caregivers operate at organizational and institutional levels. I refer to the extension of intensive prosocial caring labor outside the private sphere and into organizational and institutional arenas as "community carework."

Community carework captures the additional unpaid work caregivers do at the organizational and institutional levels, outside the home and in a variety of public settings, such as organizing educational resource fairs and fundraising events, grant writing for local nonprofit groups, advocating for school trainings, extensive group administration (i.e., maintaining email listservs, websites, and other digital resource tools), mentoring other caregivers, and volunteering at autism awareness events. Individuals rationalize their engagement in these community activities as ways to help both their own children and others. In other words, the motivation that drives participation in community carework is both self-interested and prosocial. Prosocial behaviors refer to "voluntary actions that are intended to help or benefit another individual or group of individuals" (Eisenberg & Mussen, 1989, p. 3). Accordingly, this chapter details an escalation of expert caregiving that transcends individualist boundaries and can function as an impactful prosocial force that builds community and social inclusion. At the same time, the expert caregiver toolkit continues to professionalize and challenge hierarchical bounds between lay/professional and public/private.

This chapter is the first step in thinking about carework not just as a self-interested individualistic necessity but also as a public project that deeply links the multiple worlds of caregiver self, family, and broader society. Carework conjures images that are acutely private and personal. However, my intent with community carework is to center the deep relational quality of expert caregiving that transcends the personal, intimate, private qualities that we often conjure in our minds when thinking about traditional in-home direct carework (i.e., helping loved ones with vital everyday tasks like feeding, bathing, and dressing). Instead, this chapter demonstrates how carework is fundamentally an agentic practice that affects other people, groups, and structures and therefore holds transformative power beyond the individual family.

As such, the narratives in this section expand the scope of typical direct carework and highlight the ways in which expert caregiving operates as a prosocial force for social inclusion, democratizing access to resources, and advocating for educational resources in schools. Chapter 5 expands this conceptualization of community carework further into the institutional realm by showing how systemic social change goals can be met through intensive community carework practices, and the complexities therein. Together, chapters 4 and 5 conceptualize this distinction associated with expert caregiving, which refers to the extension of caring labor outside the home and through community carework activities that bridge false dichotomies of public and private, self and society, lay and expert, and care and work.

Doing Community Carework: Extending Carework into the Local Community

All participants in this study engaged in some form of community carework, albeit levels of engagement and commitment varied widely based on one's values, time available, and personal skill set. Most (over 80 percent of the total sample) caregivers actively participated in local community-based autism education and awareness events, as either a lead organizer or a group participant, to educate the public about the diverse spectrum of autism—to put a human face to a misunderstood name. For example, many caregivers participated in family walks for autism research, volunteered at one-day community resource fairs, or organized public fundraising events to benefit local nonprofit autism support and resource groups. All caregivers described participating in at least one of these singular (one-day) events, such as a resource fair, open house at a local clinic or therapy center, or fundraising or educational event. On average, mothers participated in these events roughly once every three months.

A select number of other women (30 percent) show a higher level of commitment by assuming leadership roles in community efforts, such as spearheading local fundraising events or managing community networks. These women also often purposefully enlist their entire family's involvement in their activities. For example, Kristen works part-time as a receptionist, cares for two children ages six and four, and engages in community carework: "I'm always willing to help organizing fundraising events—creating publicity materials, soliciting donations and getting local businesses to sponsor us or donate materials. I've gotten local restaurants to provide food for free, free printing and copying of event PR stuff, free t-shirts and goodies for the kids, stuff like that. I have no problem cold-calling and going to businesses to ask for whatever we need—supplies, money, or volunteers." Therefore, Kristen's community carework involves several administrative tasks, such as organizing large public events, soliciting donations, designing and distributing publicity materials, coordinating volunteers, and general behind-the-scenes administrative work. It ebbs and flows, but roughly she spends ten hours per week on these tasks.

Community-building and social inclusion are the primary objectives that guide her motivation to engage in this administrative advocacy role. She states, "By doing this, I'm not just getting free stuff or money; I'm trying to build bridges between people, businesses, families—all of us that are living and sharing in this same community. I see it as more than just an 'autism-thing,' I'm doing something really good for my community, you know?" She continues to explain the "bigger purpose" behind her work: "Helping people in need, no matter who it is, just trying to instill this principle of community and making connections so that it's easier for people to ask for help and receive it. That's what I'm trying to do here—not just organize events or whatever." Kristen concludes by stating, "It's amazing to see how if you just ask, your local community will really step it up. It's quite moving, really. With all the battles we've fought and the bullshit we've gone through, you have absolutely no idea how much this means to me—to have a complete stranger willing to help or just be open to listening and learning about autism."

Here, she is referring to the challenges that the autistic community and their caregivers face to destigmatize autism and correct misinformation. A lot of the community work that parents do aims to challenge the monolithic and false representation of autism that circulates in the media and in dominant narratives. Autism physically and visually manifests in many different and nuanced ways. Therefore, these public events aim to show the multifaceted nature of autism, highlight the invisibility of disability, and help to minimize experiences of social exclusion. Additionally, Kristen's community carework includes a variety of unpaid professional administrative and event-planning tasks which are costly, in terms of time and money, but are important and valuable to her. Her rationale shows that for many caregivers the high costs associated with community carework, in terms of time, labor (both physical and emotional), and money, is not only self-interested but also prosocial.

Like Kristen, Laurie enjoys taking on leadership roles in organizing and planning autism awareness or resource events. She said she always gives her son Jack, eight years old, the option to attend her events or not, and frequently he likes going and meeting new people. I asked Laurie about the efficacy of her work—does tabling at farmer's markets, organizing events, making calls, and meeting with potential donors meet her goals of community building and opening up people's ideas of autism? She replied, "Yeah, I think so. Because before, we would get weird looks or people would avoid him, other kids especially, and now people make an effort to come up to us, say hi—they reach out. Kids will come up to him and say, 'Hey Jack, how are you today?' This is huge! They aren't so scared. And you should see how he [Jack] lights up." She continues, "It really makes me feel more hopeful for all of us; it's not just about me and Jack. If something was to happen and I wasn't there, I trust that someone in my neighborhood would step up and help him. And I think everyone wants to feel that way about the community that they live in, right?"

Mothers like Kristen and Laurie are actively attempting to educate and instill a sense of trust and inclusion within their local communities, through building human connections. Additionally, carework, guided by the principles of community-building, trust, and inclusivity, is a bigger project that goes beyond the direct care of one's children. In other words, the scope of community carework is far-reaching; for many mothers. taking care of their autistic children is a community project dear to their hearts, not just a personal one. Therefore, the mothers in this section demonstrate the ways that carework can expand beyond the walls of one's home and take place through a variety of different skill sets, and within diverse local public arenas.

The engagement in community carework, and the acknowledgment of a public responsibility for their work, marks a distinction associated with expert caregiving (as opposed to traditional family caregiving). Here, caregivers organize and attend events, participate in fundraising efforts for local advocacy groups, shepherd other families at the beginning of their diagnostic journeys, and manage local resources and networks to the betterment of their own children, and for others. Community carework practices are designed to help create more inclusive, informed, and supportive communities, and coordinate greater access to resources and experiential knowledge, particularly for local neurodivergent children and their families.

"I Fought and Fought and Fought": Community Carework in Schools

For parents with young children, schools are commonly a site for community carework where they sharpen their expert caregiver skills beyond the private sphere. Narratives in this section reveal the flawed structural arrangements in schools that lead (1) children with disabilities like autism to be more vulnerable to bullying in K–12 schools, and (2) caregivers to fight for accommodations and reforms. Brenna has two autistic children who have both suffered from extensive bullying in schools, not just from students but also from a teacher. Hardships in school have prompted her to secure classroom aides for both of her sons while at school, to make sure that another adult is present to witness, and prevent, any bullying situations. She states, "There have been so many complaints over the years. She [a teacher] has bullied him since first grade when he was in her class. So, he has a full-time aide. I actually have aides for both my kids. They are never alone."

Unfortunately, Brenna's story with her boys is illustrative of a situation that many families face with peer bullying. Claire also shares how her twelve-year-old son has suffered years of bullying from classmates, which came to a head with a fight in the classroom. This fight catalyzed her to take action with school administrators, which she describes here: "I went to the principal, and I told him, 'I'm sorry. I have given you so many years. You've done a great job of trying to watch this. I mean, you've hired extra people. But, look, this is ridiculous. I have to place the complaint. I have to do the safety plan.' So we filed the police report and I know he wasn't happy. We went straight to the district and filed the bullying complaint. So, they keep monitoring it and we keep going in for appointments and meetings and stuff like that." A school safety plan is an official document designed to address specific behaviors that may be harmful to the student or to others. It formalizes a plan, with support, if the student exhibits unsafe behavior to keep all students safe.

Claire has worked tirelessly as an advocate for her son particularly in the school system, volunteering with the special education board and actively participating in education-based advocacy workshops and events. She has independently educated herself on all the current laws and regulations, specific to the state of California and her local school district, regarding special education and disability rights in education. She parlays this knowledge and education into action on behalf of her child in school. She acknowledges how this process of translating knowledge and skills into empirical action can be empowering; she sees herself as a force to be reckoned with and taken seriously by school authority figures and administrators. Claire states, "I think it took our principal two or three years to realize that I work a lot with the district, and I know what I'm talking about with special ed and what my kids deserve in the classroom and what should not be happening in school." "I think he played me for a fool a little bit, like I wouldn't do anything about the bullying, that he didn't need to take me seriously. It wasn't easy, but I followed through with every complaint and filed every document and contacted every person that I needed to," she adds.

"He played me for a fool a little bit" harkens back to the diagnostic journey for many mothers who struggled with instances of dismissal or delegitimization from medical authorities. Pushing back against institutional authorities is a part of expert caregiving, which is learned over time and does not come easily to most. However, some caregivers like Claire continue to overcome significant institutional barriers with impressive results.

This chapter opened with Fiona and her family. Fiona also provides an impressive example of community carework, as she has advocated on behalf of her children for accommodations in the classroom and fought for mandatory autism training for all school faculty in her sons' elementary school. With much pride and a sense of accomplishment, she states, "And I fought and fought and fought, to get them training. The entire school got autism training two weeks ago and I was there. It was quite a moment for me." The training focused on educating faculty about autism and effective accommodations in the classroom for autistic students. The program was so successful that she was confident it would be extended to teachers and administrators in other schools in the district.

Fiona continued to emphasize the efficacy of the training to educate and increase teachers' understanding of autism and improve the experiences of autistic children in school: "After, I had teachers come up to me and tell me, 'I thought I knew autism.' One of them particularly, she goes, 'I thought I knew it. But I didn't. I'm around your son all the time, and I had no idea about half of it.'" Therefore, Fiona is a lay caregiver who single-handedly instituted a mandatory autism education program for all faculty in a public school, which proved to be effective and useful. Further, the intent with the training is to help facilitate a more positive, inclusive learning environment for all children, and especially those with disabilities. Therefore, Fiona's work here has the potential to improve not only her own sons' experiences at school but also the experiences of many other children who need accommodations in the classroom. It is important to note here that while Fiona has achieved significant results in her sons' school, her practices are very much rooted in advocating for her own children, with secondary benefits for others; her orientation to advocacy and structural change is limited in scope. However, she demonstrates a potential of community carework to promote social inclusion and neurodiversity-affirming accommodations within local public schools.

Therefore, in this section we see varying levels of engagement and forms of community carework that have the potential to influence more than just a single child or family, classroom, or neighborhood. Organizing fundraising events, securing training for school staff, maintaining email listservs, and coordinating resource networks are examples of ways expert caregiving continues to intensify and expand into the public sphere. Through community carework, mothers take on additional professional roles as public health educator, event planner and fundraiser, publicity manager, disability advocate, and more, with significant impact on one's local community.

The intensification of carework into these public realms highlights the existing flaws or gaps therein for autistic children and their families. For example, advocacy in schools would not be needed if teachers received training in neurodiversity-affirming methods to support neurodiverse learners in the classroom. If the diagnostic process and support therapies were accessible and streamlined, resource sharing and network building would not be so vital. If local autism community organizations or nonprofit support services were adequately funded, caregiver-led grant writing and fundraising efforts would not have to be a priority. Therefore, community carework is a useful way to highlight gaps in existing care systems that drive the intensification of carework—individual caregivers are left to fill these meso-level holes.

By demonstrating the pro–social advocacy practices associated with community carework, this chapter builds on existing literature on intensive motherhood and ways that negotiating and securing resources have increasingly come under the purview of what it means to be a "good mother." Specifically, sociologist Jaqueline Litt (2004) created the concept of "advocacy care work" to account for work that extends beyond the direct care of a child (i.e., feeding, bathing, and disciplining), which "attempts to create resources, recapture resources that had been lost, and/or correct for [problems in] those services currently at hand" (p. 628). In her work, advocacy carework takes the form of lengthy negotiations with schools, insurance companies, and other daily tasks necessary to secure resources. Kibria and Suarez Becerra (2021) offer the concept of the "Good Advocate Mother" to capture the interplay between race, immigration, and expanding cultural expectations of good mothering when navigating special education systems in the United States. Additionally, Linda Blum (2007) refers to mothers like the ones featured in this chapter as "vigilantes," who "seize authority . . . within educational and medical systems in the midst of turf wars, cost containment, and a resulting proliferation of medication treatments" (p. 202).

Building on this literature, I offer the concept of community carework as a prosocial extension of existing advocacy carework concepts that are primarily individualistic and self/child-interested. In other words, existing concepts are primarily motivated by and focus on one's personal interest, usually to gain access to resources in formal systems to benefit their own children. With community carework, caregivers broaden the scope of both their motivation and impact to benefit not just their child but also their local community, and for some, this extends further to include engagement with larger structures beyond the local. In doing so, community carework is a set of practices that is both self-interested and prosocial and can have positive impact on multiple scales—the micro (individual), meso (community), and macro (systems) levels. Additionally, community carework often involves individual risk for collective gain, which is exemplified in chapter 5. In conceptualizing community carework as a turn away from primarily individualist rationales and traditional direct care practices, we can see how carework can operate as an important ground for community building, social inclusion, and social change.

Although the above narratives show concrete patterns in the intensification and translation of autism carework into the public realm through prosocial community carework, this does not mean that all caregivers engage in these practices in the same way, nor do they all express the same motivation or goals. The different rationales that guide community carework practices in this chapter are heightened when calls for more direct action push their public work onto the political stage. Expanding the scale and scope of community carework practices to include intensive institutional engagement is a major point of contention within the autism caregiver community, which is explored in chapter 5.

5
Potentials and Limits of Expert Caregiving
Community Carework and Medicalization

I met Amy, an emergency room physician and mother of two autistic boys ages eleven and fourteen, for a chat outside a coffee shop one Saturday afternoon. I ordered coffee for both of us and settled in at a table outside in the warm spring sunshine. Amy bustled over, took off her jacket, and greeted me with a smile, eager to tell her story. "Let's get to it, yeah I have two hours and a lot to say!" she said with enthusiasm in her voice.

In addition to the administrative and educational advocacy work that the mothers in chapter 4 described, Amy extends her community carework to the political stage through direct action mechanisms geared at structural change. She describes one of her proudest moments in which she "organized hundreds of autistic people and their families to gather on the steps of the state capitol in Sacramento in protest of various proposed cuts to developmental services and new special ed policies that will drastically harm our kids." I asked her to explain a bit more about what she did regarding this event, and she replied, "I helped transport people and encouraged them to testify at a hearing and follow up with local legislators. It's really rewarding to see hundreds of children and their families sharing their stories in support of the same cause."

This chapter builds on chapter 4's account of the extension of expert caregiving into the public sphere through community carework for social inclusion, community building, and educational advocacy. Although meaningful and important, prosocial practices are limited in scope and intensity of influence and involve relatively low risks for the caregiver. Instead, this chapter details an escalation of the prosocial turn in carework practices that maximizes the potential for expert caregiving to operate as a transformative public project. Here, the rationales that guide heightened engagement at the institutional level include a desire to shift the paradigms through which we culturally understand autism (from private to public) and explicitly address the flaws in care systems dedicated to autistic and neurodivergent communities. The mechanisms of community carework in this section are oriented toward collective, systemic change with the potential for wide-scale benefit, which oftentimes comes with a cost for individuals.

Further, in the attempt to call out problems in dominant medical, education, and cultural systems and actively work to change them, significant tensions and divisions arise within the caregiver community. Accordingly, this chapter also demonstrates key factors that constrain the practice of expert carework as a transformative public project, which include private versus public models for understanding autism and the "double-edged sword" of medicalization.

"At Least for Me, I Feel a Bigger Responsibility": Transformative Potentials of Community Carework

Some mothers feel a duty to maximize their carework by engaging extensively and regularly at the level of institutions. In this case, institutional engagement refers to the extension of caring labor to the realm of education, health care, and politics, and demands change. In doing so, community carework publicizes caregiver grievances and needs, and works toward reforming institutional policy or structural arrangements. For example, like Amy, some mothers organize rallies to protest educational policies or lead letter-writing campaigns to local legislators, and in doing so, their community carework operates as a structural social change mechanism. They see their carework as a form of political critique and mechanism for change, not just for their child, but to benefit all of us. The narratives in this section shed light on individual motivations, practices, and potentials for community carework to facilitate large structural changes.

For example, Isabel is a stay-at-home mother who described political organizing and campaign work as a prime component of her community carework: "I call it my 'second job.'" I say that because I really treat it like a job. I take it very seriously; I'm hardworking and organized and dedicated." Isabel has a bachelor's degree in marketing and used to work in a large corporation before having children, so she brings her business skills into her community carework. She is adept at mobilizing resources and people in her community. Her work not only is administrative or educational but also supports a reform agenda by actively and consistently engaging in political work that targets structural change. For example, she states, "I've created these lengthy listservs for all community contacts, I have spreadsheets that keep track of all the proposed policy changes and legislative measures on the docket, and then I organize tabling events at local grocery stores, farmers markets, outside my kids' schools, coffee shops—wherever! I send out major email blasts to over 1,000 community members—both in the autism community and not—soliciting volunteers for events or to ask them to write or call local politicians."

Studies of parental disability activism, such as Allison Carey, Pamela Block, & Richard Scotch's (2020) *Allies and Obstacles*, show the complexities associated with parent- or caregiver-led activism, and the historical tensions between disability activists and parents of disabled children. Parental activism is not the central focus of this study, as only a minority of women in this sample actively worked toward politicizing autism and autism carework. Although they are a minority in numbers, their impact is substantial and worthy of discussion, particularly because they highlight the potential and tensions associated with extending carework into political realms.

Additionally, Leah, a part-time administrative assistant with a bachelor's degree and mother of a four-year-old autistic daughter, explains the "bigger things" that guide her community carework: "I'm involved in my local autism groups so I can help connect new families or tell them about my experiences. Basically, to answer the questions that no one else seems able to do, or doesn't want to. But, I'm really talking about the bigger things here—we need to write to legislators, start petitions, go to your local school board, attend every meeting; you can call up local government officers so they do not forget about us! I've seen it work. If you keep the heat on them, if they know that you are watching them, change happens and it's exciting and rewarding." Here, Leah and Isabel represent a particular form of community carework that is geared toward social and political change through institutional reforms, primarily in education and health care. Beyond simply lending administrative support, these caregivers engage in direct-action social change measures, such as disseminating information to the public, engaging with local media, organizing political campaigns, circulating petitions and calls for action, and participating in rallies and protests primarily calling for reforms in education. They see their work as purposeful and necessary, and as a large part of who they are as mothers, women, and community members. Carework that has explicit structural change goals, be it in education or health care, has the potential to impact a much bigger audience that cuts across neurotypical-neurodivergent lines.

Rachel expresses the same sentiment, as she "can't just sit around and do nothing, when there is so much that needs to be done not just in our daily lives, but I mean big changes." These big changes include "the whole IEP [independent education plan] system for kids in schools. . . . There are so many problems and so much red tape." She then proceeded to tell me about her first time trying to navigate the IEP process for her son, which amplifies the ways structural flaws create an isolated, stressful, individualized caring experience. She states, "Oh, and you know, the first time I had to complete all of this paperwork for his IEP and the schools, I had no idea what I was doing; I was a mess about it."

"What did you do?" I asked. She replied, "So, I brought all the forms with me to a support group meeting and pretty much begged someone to help me. So, another parent, pretty much a stranger, sat down with me for almost two hours and walked me through the forms and answered my thousands of questions. Can you believe that? And I know I'm not the only one who has dealt with this; we need to make some real systematic changes to help our community out, and I'm taking this on!" Informed by her early experiences, Rachel has joined her local school board to be an agent of "big change" particularly in schools. Therefore, Rachel exemplifies some of the structural roots and personal grievances that often motivate caregivers to dedicate their community carework toward making "big changes."

The intensive community carework highlighted in this section by mothers like Leah and Isabel functions as a form of collective agency aimed at structural change and policy reform that aligns with the social model of autism. For example, Leah demonstrates the ways in which community carework can operate as a means to subvert the dominance of the biomedical model of autism and promote neurodiversity. With passion, she states, "We need bigger changes in education, in medicine, and scientific research. Enough with this 'Autism is a disease that we need to cure' crap! You would die if you knew how much money goes into finding a cure for autism. It's such B.S.! All that money and scientific brilliance should be spent getting families connected with the resources that they actually need, not a 'cure.'"

We have seen how some caregivers consciously incorporate a bigger project of challenging the biomedical model in their everyday carework, with tangible successes. They understand autism not as a disease to be cured, but instead as a neurotype and disability that deserves social reforms, accommodations, and inclusion. For example, Leah is highly critical of the cure focus, Amy works to replace ABA techniques with neurodiversity-affirming interventions in schools, and many others critique the delayed and flawed diagnostic process that requires changes in health care. In these everyday actions, especially in health care and education, mothers' experiential knowledge is going head-to-head with institutional dogma. In doing so, mothers are challenging the top-down hierarchical knowledge and power relations inherent within the organization of traditional institutions like medicine.

Specifically, when mothers push back, follow up, fight, call and call again, and demand meetings or revised reports, status inequalities are challenged between doctor and patient/caregiver, student/teacher, and parent/principal. In other words, the extension of expert carework into formal institutional spheres has the potential to subvert traditional power dynamics, and specifically to elevate the status and power of lay, lived, experiential knowledge. In doing so, I conceptualize the expert caregiver as an agent of change who can exert power against institutions with the goal of shaping them to match their lived realities.

The narratives in this section detail the maximization of community carework and shed light on the motivation for stepping up unpaid care practices and politicizing autism carework. However, not all caregivers desire to engage extensively in the political public realm or incorporate these values into their own self-identity. The following section details tensions that surround the use of carework for systemic change, which highlights important obstacles to the transformative power of carework.

Detaching from the "Nutty, Pushy Kind": Limits to Community Carework

Not all caregivers desired to engage in intensive community carework, and many expressed uneasiness and discomfort with anything that they perceived as political or activist in nature. Specifically, more than half of the caregivers in this sample expressed fears of being labeled a "pushy parent," because of their "outspokenness" in their work to secure services, rights, and care. For example, Beth describes her fear of being one of those "pushy parents": "I don't think of myself as an advocate, really. I tend to be a people pleaser, and the label 'advocate' is more the nutty, pushy kind, although I suppose I don't let anyone tell me no. Just if there's something that might help, I expect to be allowed to try it, and if it doesn't work, I'm always the first to say, 'Okay. My bad.'" (She makes the hands-up gesture.)

Others exhibited similarly cautious approaches to community carework. For example, Yvette describes herself as an active "audience member," who is happy to show her support and attend events but prefers not to get involved any further. Here, she explains the rationale behind her position as an "audience member," "I like to call myself an 'audience member' at these autism events and stuff. I do go to things; it's just I don't like to get too involved." I asked, "Why?" To which she replied, "For one thing, I don't really have the time. I work part-time and I take care of three kids, one of whom is autistic, which is a full-time job in itself. So, honestly, any extra time I have is not spent organizing things or protesting or petitioning, you know what I mean? Who has time for this?" She continues, "And secondly, I don't want to get the reputation as one of those confrontational pushy parents. I kind of hate those people—too aggressive—so I really don't want to be grouped in as one of them. So, I go to events to keep informed about everything, but I keep to myself more as an audience member and less as leader."

Additionally, Joanne describes how publicizing her experiences could threaten important relationships and resources. She fears that in becoming "too vocal" or "too political" she may lose the crucial support of family members, friends, her case worker, or doctors. She states, "Sometimes, I think I should be doing more. I have a friend who is active politically—she goes and talks to local governors and school administrators and cold-calls people. I always sign the petition, send the emails, but I do get scared to put my name on things or get too active, too vocal, too out-there, you know?" I asked her what she was scared about. She sighed and then said, "I think I'm just really scared to rock the boat, like we have gone through so much to get the mix of people, therapies, doctors that we have, and I'm simply not willing to risk any of it. Each one of these pieces is vital—our babysitter, lawyer, neurologist, pediatrician, nutritionist, even my family and husband's parents—we desperately need the support and help from all of these people, and you never know who may not agree with your politics and cut you off, or see you as liability or something. I just can't do that to my family." Joanne was visibly worried as she thought about potentially jeopardizing her current care team; I could see the fear in her eyes as she spoke. These very real fears reflect the inaccessibility of vital care services that caregivers have fought so hard to secure.

Similarly, Stephanie is very close with her extended family and relies on her parents to help with childcare. She explains how her upbringing and practical time-management issues are key limits to her community carework: "I was always raised to not rock the boat; my parents instilled that in me. Social justice and political stuff was never something that I'm interested in or encouraged to do." She continues, "If my parents—who are retired and watch my kids two days a week—or husband knew I was using my free time to get involved in activist stuff, they definitely would not be supportive, and honestly, I don't think it's the best use of my time either. I say leave that up to people who are good at it! I don't think that's me." Here, Stephanie also articulates how fears and hesitancies that surround "not rocking the boat" or being the "pushy parent" are gendered and informed by early gender socialization.

"Pushy," "bossy," and "assertive" are adjectives that carry gender connotations and are often used when women deviate from cultural norms of femininity. Oftentimes, speaking up to advocate for one's child, challenging authority figures (especially men), and fighting for structural reforms in public arenas violate many of the societal expectations deemed appropriate for women and the role of mothers. In several cases, the pressure from family members to disengage in this type of work is gendered not only because it violates traditional gender norms for women but also because it may be seen as a threat to mothers' ability to fulfill their role in the domestic sphere. Extensive community carework is labor intensive and requires expending a lot of time and energy outside the home and family, time and energy that otherwise may be spent at home fulfilling familial and household responsibilities. Accordingly, narrative descriptions that reference "pushy" or "nut" parents illuminate how persistent gender and traditional nuclear family norms can limit community carework.

Therefore, narratives in this section provide insight into why only a minority of caregivers center their community carework on identifying structural issues and actively working to change them through public political avenues. They describe very realistic constraints to engaging in extensive community carework, which include time-management, family responsibilities, gendered pressures from family members, and fears of losing their hard-won support team and safety net. In these ways, we see how individual carework can exist in conflict with community carework, and the tensions that exist between individual needs and community needs. Most mothers simply do not have the time to get involved in activities that exceed the direct care of their child and household; being an "audience member" is as close as it gets to front-line social change participation. Few are actually standing on the steps of the capitol protesting educational reforms or calling for changes in health care, but some are.

Most women in this sample live in relatively privileged social locations, primarily advantaged by race and class, which affords greater access to resources like money, time, social capital, education, and professional skills: money to pay out-of-pocket expenses to support fundraising efforts or guest speakers, time to attend rallies or school board meetings, and the skill to write emails and design PR materials. They have social connections with influential community members to help publicize an event, meet with a potential large donor, or secure a meeting with a local politician. Their professional skills, a result of high levels of educational attainment, allow some to navigate disability laws and others to lead workshops on how to advocate for their children in the IEP process with schools. Access to these resources allows mothers to expand their circle of influence and increase the breadth of their community carework.

At the same time, many others caring for autistic children do not have the luxuries of time, dense social networks, or professional skills to transfer into their carework. Further, this type of community work necessitates a level of comfortability working within institutions and with the public. Especially non-native English speakers, mixed-status families, and historically disadvantaged families of color may have a harder time doing this type of carework or may be completely disinterested in doing so at all because of a lack of trust with authority figures and institutions. For undocumented or mixed-status families and families of color, any involvement with institutions and formal bureaucracies is a risky endeavor that can pose a threat to their families and their vital support network.

Many mothers fear that a "pushy parent," one who is more vocal and politically active, may sacrifice existing resources, services, and social ties, for which they have already fought tirelessly. Joanne expressed how she is not willing to compromise the resources, family, and professional support that she has amassed so far for the purpose of getting involved in direct-action measures. To these mothers, the possibilities of direct action are too risky; they are not willing to risk "burning bridges" with specialists whom they have waited to see for over a year or endangering a good working relationship with a caseworker, teacher, or family member. These fears are completely understandable given the battles families have waged to secure resources—it is risky. More importantly, these very real fears and motivations are significant obstacles to challenging the medicalization of autism and to shifting the paradigm from understanding it as a private, individual biomedical disease to a social disability and a difference in neurotype.

"It's Family Business": Limits to Community Carework

In this section, I offer an additional way to understand the hesitancy to maximize the practice of community carework, which is grounded in private orientations of autism and medicalization. Here, caregivers reveal how their fundamental orientation to autism and the social caring experience can either obstruct or promote the transformative power of carework for individuals and society. According to Peter Conrad (1992), medicalization occurs on three levels: "a problem is defined in medical terms, using medical language; understood through the adoption of a medical framework; 'treated' with medical intervention" (p. 211). Every family in this study has actively fought to have their child's behaviors medicalized to receive a diagnosis and continue to engage in a series of medical interventions. Many parents who have fought tirelessly for medical recognition, an official diagnosis, and quality care see activism as a threat to the medicalization of autism and accordant support services.

Community carework that targets structural changes and includes political engagement challenges the medicalization of autism as a purely private and personal experience between individual families and medical professionals. How individual caregivers make sense of autism and their caring experiences guide their carework, and especially the extent to which they engage outside the home. Therefore, this section features some of the caregivers who represent a private understanding of autism as something personal, as opposed to public, and managed within the family as directed by medical professionals, as opposed to a collective experience of disability. Accordingly, the voices in this section provide insight into the constraints associated with community carework and the limits to carework as a transformative project and force for change.

Anne's family represents the inclination to privatize family experiences of autism, which limits her engagement in community carework: "I see some of these parents on TV and at events and it is just not me. I remember one day, while I was sitting in bed next to my stack of ten autism books reading away, my husband turned to me and said, 'Just promise me you'll never become one of those crazy autism moms that we saw on TV today. It's a family issue, not something to go on TV about.'" She continues to describe autism carework as "family business" that is managed within the home and directed by her son's doctors and therapists, "not something to go on TV to talk about with the world and strangers!"

Similarly, Maria describes how her family negotiated their decision to keep life as "normal as possible" by keeping autism carework in-home and within the family. She states, "It was a long process, but long ago, as a family we decided the top priority was keeping life as normal as possible for all of us. I don't do any of the activist stuff that I hear other people do, because I wouldn't do it for my other kids, and I want to treat everyone the same way. We kind of block out all that other stuff. We just stay out of all of the autism, vaccine debates stuff that you see on TV and read about. . . . Keep it simple!"

Others described "not feeling comfortable announcing private material to the world" and a general uneasiness with disclosing "family business," as Karen states: "I don't think I need to put it all out there, you know?" We hear in the words above a clear uneasiness and discomfort talking about autism, and a strategic distancing away from intensive community carework. For some, the desire to be tight-lipped and very private about their carework may be informed by the emotion of shame, particularly contextualized within an ableist society. Shame can emerge when an individual deviates from social norms and is judged harshly by others for doing so.

As demonstrated in chapter 2, reoccurring experiences of social exclusion, familial tensions, and "bad mother stares" due to deviating from neurotypical norms can be internalized and manifest in uncomfortable self-feelings of shame that dramatically impact one's identity. Psychologists John Terrizzi and Natalie Shook (2020) explain the relationship between shame and the self: "The experience of shame encourages self-evaluative ruminations that are degrading and pervade all aspects of the self (i.e., both physical and psychological). As such, the self is perceived as innately flawed. Thus, shame is a negatively valenced self-conscious emotion that results in global self-condemnation." Accordingly, feelings of shame can be a force that drives the privatization of the autism caring experience and limits the transformative potentials of community carework.

Additionally, a private framework of autism aligns with the dominant biomedical paradigm. By operating purely within the private biomedical paradigm, autism is practiced as an individual disease or disorder, not a social disability. Accordingly, this subset of caregivers can be understood as lay agents of medicalization who follow the biomedical model of disease and hierarchical doctor-patient relationships.

This private, biomedical interpretation means that the power to conceptualize, diagnose, and treat "nonnormative" bodies and minds remains in the hands of medical professionals and is organized within the healthcare system, which limits possibilities for alternative understandings of normality and frameworks of disability. Simply put, private orientations obstruct the larger cultural project to shift the paradigm on autism. Further, intensive community carework, particularly aimed at structural change and political engagement, does not align with such a model—it doesn't make sense.

The Messiness of Medicalization

On the other hand, disability frameworks that support demedicalization afford individuals greater autonomy and can help blur the medical gaze by affording nonmedical entities power and legitimacy in labeling, framing, and treating autism as a social disability. According to Conrad (1992), demedicalization refers to "a problem that no longer retains its medical definition" (p. 224). Such demedicalizing practices would facilitate a conceptual shift in the way in which autism is understood, from the isolated individual body/mind to the surrounding social environment; not only to examine what is going on *within* one human body, but to consider what is happening *around* that child to understand lived experiences. Demedicalizing practices extend authority to caregivers' experiential knowledge, and in doing so, may help to curb the deference to medical professionals. In other words, instead of deferring completely to professionals, caregivers learn to trust themselves and the knowledge gained through living as an expert caregiver.

Community carework that centers political engagement for social change works to demedicalize autism and the autism caring experience. As demonstrated in the caring practices of Leah, Isabel, and Amy, their efforts work to normalize autism as an accepted neurological difference, as opposed to a private disease or an abnormal disorder. Further, their work securely places autism discussions and actions outside of just medicine and health care. The primary goals of political engagement practices include school reforms, funding for local community groups, and public awareness; they are not simply advocating for better access to health care or more affordable therapeutic services. Instead, autism and autism carework are framed as a public concern particularly regarding education and school services and social inclusion and ideas of normality. In doing so, autism is taken outside the strict jurisdiction of medicine and the individual biological body, thereby challenging its medicalization and expanding the scope and scale of typical carework.

That said, even exemplars of community carework rooted in the social model of disability fought to have their children medically diagnosed, which is a point not taken lightly. This shows the messiness of the medicalization process involved in lived experiences of neurodivergence and disability. For example, in studies of fibromyalgia support groups, Kristin Barker (2005, 2008) found an important paradox inherent within medical consumerism and the process of lay challenge to medical authority, in which "challenges to medical authority and demands for medicalization become one" (p. 17); also referred to as a "double-edged sword" (1983) by Catherine Riessman, who has written extensively on the ways medicalization is used as a means for social control in women's lives. Similarly, in Laura Mauldin's (2016) research on cochlear implant technology and their complex impacts on deaf children and deaf culture, she found that families experienced "ambivalent medicalization," which emphasizes how people are "both empowered by and surrendering to the process of medicalization" (p. 4). Mauldin (2016) argues that the process of medicalization is in and of itself ambivalent—mixed and contradictory—with good and bad aspects.

My research fits this interesting puzzle. A subset of caregivers fights for medical recognition, surveillance, and care and prioritize lay experiential knowledge and institutional reforms that challenge the authority of medical professionals and formal institutions.

In this sense, lay caregivers pose as both agents of medicalization and threats to the authority of medicalization; they help to broaden the jurisdiction of medicine while also challenging top-down medical expertise and the formal healthcare system.

The paradox here is striking. In the attempt to secure services, enact policy reforms, challenge dominant lay/expert knowledge production, and increase public awareness of autism as a disability, not a disease, caregivers are simultaneously enabling and challenging medicalization. Caregivers and patients absolutely need formal medical recognition and diagnosis to receive life-altering services and rights, but in doing so they actively expand the jurisdiction of medicine into individual family life and direct care of children, as well as into macro-level educational programming, school policy reforms, and broader national legislation. If an official medical diagnosis remains as a gatekeeper to vital services and rights, this tension will remain. More importantly, this ambivalence toward medicalization serves as a formidable limit to shifting cultural understandings of autism and challenging biomedical dominance.

The narratives in this section highlight the tensions within community carework as a public project. These tensions reside in the juxtaposition of carework for building community, challenging top-down medical authority, and advocating for significant social reforms, with the desire to maintain vital healthcare resources and social support networks. For many, they seem to be walking a tightrope between staying within the boundaries deemed appropriate as lay caregiver and mother and pushing these borders to advocate for educational reforms and maximize access to healthcare services. The equilibrium of this tightrope is unique to each caregiver's preferences and skill sets, though together they demonstrate important limits and possibilities for community carework at large.

Care work often activates those who had been previously politically inactive citizens, expanding their boundaries because of the care they provide for their families. In fact, feminist analyses of citizenship have made it clear that women's care work often stimulates women's political activity (Herd & Meyer, 2002, p. 672).

In this chapter, we see how the motivation behind many mothers' community carework is differently oriented and larger in both scope and scale. Caregivers are not simply building community in the service of their child; instead, their carework occurs within a politicized, public realm, manifested in organizing protests on the steps of the state capitol and testifying at hearings to actively work toward systemic changes, all of which significantly expand definitions of typical direct carework.

In chapter 4, I introduced the concept of "community carework" to name the meso-level forms and spaces in which expert caregivers labor, additionally, outside the home both for their own families and for others. A distinct quality associated with expert caregiving is this engagement in community carework that can range from minor behind-the-scenes administrative and coordination work to educational advocacy and committed efforts to support structural changes in health care and education. In doing so, autism carework becomes a public project strategically designed to address structural flaws in education, health care, and ableist cultural norms.

Together, these different dimensions and public pathways of caregiving extend caring labor into the local community to help other children and families navigate healthcare and educational bureaucracies, change public attitudes or misinformation about autism, institute policy and programmatic reforms, and reform the overall climate in schools so that all children are included and supported in their learning. Community carework functions to strengthen the connections between individuals, local communities, and broader society and to build stronger safety nets to support isolated individual caregivers.

Further, community carework practices and rationales exist on a wide-ranging spectrum. On the one hand, some mothers' carework demands structural change and exists as a challenge to authoritative traditional institutions like medicine and education. Others express great fear of being seen as one of these "nutty" or "pushy" parents who operate purposefully within the public, political sphere. Many fall in between these two poles. Most mothers engage in administrative and educational community carework practices, in which they work hard to build community resources for local neurodivergent children and their families but do not engage in direct action or spearhead educational reforms. Constraints to the expanse of community carework to the political stage include time management and trying to balance work-family responsibilities, gendered pressures from family members to avoid politics, and fears of losing vital support services. Being "too vocal," "too pushy," or "too demanding" is perceived by some as a threat to a family's current treatment plan and support network, which most families are unwilling to risk. To these mothers, the possibilities of any political engagement or politicizing their own identities is too risky, providing insight into the constraints associated with collective action and mobilization for any health, illness, or disability cause.

Further, in this chapter we see the ways in which the competing models of autism—private/biomedical and public/social—are embedded into actual carework practices, with vastly different results. Particularly when caregivers asked to push their carework onto the political stage and engage in structural critique or change, the hegemony of the private biomedical framework of autism becomes more apparent. Further, the uneasiness with structural critique and political engagement and the general hesitancy to publicize autism-related experiences constrain the extent to which caregivers participate in community carework and expose important barriers to the transformative power of carework.

The extension of carework into formal institutional spheres has the potential to subvert traditional power dynamics, and specifically to elevate the status and power of lay experiential knowledge. Accordingly, expert caregivers engaged in a variety of forms of carework possess the power to bridge false dichotomies of public and private, self and society, lay and professional, and unpaid care and paid work.

6
"I Need Some Air Down Here and Nobody Is Noticing"
Caring about the Expert Caregiver

> I'll leave you with this analogy. I feel like I'm standing in quicksand and I'm holding my kids up over my head and I'm pushing them upward, and making sure that they're OK, and I'm sinking, but nobody notices. That's kind of exactly what I feel like, you know what I mean? I need some air down here and nobody is noticing.

This image that Candace provides above is a compelling illustration of the invisibility of carework and its unseen impacts on caregivers. The cumulative responsibilities, expanding roles, conflicting demands, and feelings of isolation that are a part of contemporary expert caregiving take a toll on caregivers, especially if their work is seldom acknowledged. There are few moments or areas in caregivers' daily lives that caring does not touch, and they need support, though few come out and say it. If caregivers are struggling and unable to care for themselves, they have no care to give (to their children, families, and communities). In the feminist ethic of care tradition, it is prudent to take carework seriously because it is the bedrock of healthy social relationships and thriving families and societies.

As political theorist Joan Tronto (1993) states, "On the most general level, we suggest that caring be viewed as a species activity that includes everything that we do to maintain, continue, and repair our 'world' so that we can live in it as well as possible. That world includes our bodies, ourselves, and our environment, all of which we seek to interweave in a complex, life-sustaining web" (p. 103). Accordingly, expert caregiving includes a set of daily mechanisms that allow children to thrive for the betterment of us all, and within a world that is not particularly designed for them. This means that children with disabilities (and their caregivers and families) experience challenges and hardships (i.e., social exclusion, stigma, and discrimination) that able-bodied and neurotypical people do not. It is simply harder to navigate a world whose institutions are not designed on your strengths, and whose ingrained cultural assumptions and expectations are contrary to your existence. The process of becoming an expert caregiver spotlights complex, and at times contradictory, relationships among nurturant carework, gender, family, and medicalization and exposes structural flaws in "the rest of the world."

Paradox One: Expert Caregiving, Gender, and Family Inequalities

Narratives in this case study demonstrate deep, complex relationships among nurturant carework, gender, and the family. More specifically, the process of becoming an expert caregiver shows the conditions that both enable and constrain women's ability to challenge the normative gender structure through carework. Expert caregiving can paradoxically undermine cultural expectations for women and care as a feminine project, while also upholding a strict gendered division of labor at home and in society.

This book adds new dimensions to existing conceptualizations of "intensive mothering" (Hays, 1996), "concerted cultivation" (Lareau, 2011), "Vigilante Mothers" (Blum, 2007, 2015), "intensive feeding ideology" (Brenton, 2017), and "advocacy care work" (Litt, 2004) to include social actions and roles that challenge cisgender norms for women and confines of the feminine domestic caring sphere. Expert caregiving expands the jurisdiction of unpaid carework past the feminine sphere to include active participation in formal paternalistic institutions of science, medicine and health care, education, and politics, all of which are a part of the traditionally masculine public sphere.

Andrea Miller and Eugene Bogida (2016) define separate spheres ideology as a "belief system that claims that: 1) gender differences in society are innate, rather than culturally or situationally created; 2) these innate differences lead men and women to freely participate in different spheres of society; and 3) gendered differences in participation in public and private spheres are natural, inevitable, and desirable" (p. 2). Therefore, women are expected to be responsible for the domestic sphere—anything care-oriented that occurs within the home and family—and a man's place is outside the home in public institutional arenas, and this binary gendered division of social life is naturalized. Importantly, as Celia Davies (1995) notes, "the public world, or at least the masculinist fiction of it, is devoid of caring. Culturally, it is built on this absence, it celebrates it" (p. 24).

Therefore, when expert caregivers incorporate the following behaviors and skills into their everyday lives, they are actively pushing the confines of separate spheres and the normative gender structure: scientific observation and analysis, diagnostic tracking of behaviors, therapeutic protocol design, medicalese and health literacy, navigating bureaucratic health care systems, specialized knowledge and modalities specific to PT, OT, and speech therapy, and community carework skills like lobbying for educational or healthcare reforms and advocating for institutional changes.

By practicing new skills, bodies of knowledge, and agentic interactions with authority figures, caregivers work to overcome institutional obstacles in the caring experience, while also pushing the strict bounds of traditional gender roles and separate spheres ideology that promote gender inequality. In doing so, lay women gain access to decision-making power and important resources that are empowering and can minimize experiences of subordination within institutions like the family, health care, and education.

While expert caregiving can be empowering, or perhaps emancipatory in moments for some, it can also be constraining for women. Feminists argue that the family mediates the relationship between individuals and society, reflects broader hierarchical social arrangements, and can serve as an arm of patriarchy. This means that the social organization within a private family can uphold unequal and oppressive societal arrangements and gender ideologies.

Expert carework can be all consuming, and for many women this means that much of their life is centered around the traditionally feminine act of carework. Expert caregiving expands the responsibilities, spheres of engagement, and costs for lay caregivers exponentially, which frequently constrains women's ability to be or do anything else. In chapter 2, we see clearly how many mothers experience psychological distress and mental health struggles due to the overwhelming demands associated with both the unequal division of carework at home and paid work. There is simply not enough time in the day to be an expert caregiver, excel professionally, engage in hobbies, maintain a home, marriage, and family, and meet any other external commitments, without help. Instead, women make sacrifices in their careers and personal life outside the home to prioritize their caretaking responsibilities, in alignment with traditional gender roles for women and ideals of good mothers. In doing so, the focus of women's lives is centered within the traditional domestic sphere and on family and caregiving. For many, this shift has a profoundly destabilizing effect on their self-identity.

Most women in this study experienced strained social relationships, job loss, or trouble finding flexible work that allowed them to balance work and family caregiving. They made certain sacrifices that, in most cases, their husbands did not, and rarely were they negotiated or discussed. Instead, women were expected and assumed to make these sacrifices in the public-facing aspects of their life (largely in their careers), which reflects the entrenched nature of gender traditionalism and the persistent power of the separate spheres ideology. Further, especially in the cases of women who left the paid labor force (either by choice or by force), the gendered expectations associated with expert caregiving can facilitate lasting gender inequalities. Without the ability to be financially self-sufficient, traditional gendered power dynamics persist within the private and public spheres that can significantly constrain women's agency.

Additionally, cultural ideals of the American family and "good mothering" uphold unrealistic expectations for women that shape the caregiving experience and uphold broader unequal societal arrangements that constrain women's agency. Overwhelmingly, mothers feel that they have nowhere and no one to turn to for help, because doing anything differently would be a violation of "good mothering" that comes with social costs. Without clear answers, accessible resources, and systems of support to help mothers and families, individually they shoulder the ever-growing carework load, largely silently and invisibly. In this way, expert carework can function to maintain the gender hierarchy and hegemonic ideals of the traditional nuclear family, which includes very precise and unrealistic expectations for mothers.

Paradoxically, expert caregiving also is a mechanism to subvert systemic inequalities in everyday pragmatic ways. Specifically, together the chapters in this book show how expert carework operates as a set of strategic practices that hold the power to challenge structural inequalities and allow caregivers to assert their agency in shaping both their lived experiences and dominant systems even in the smallest ways, and in the places and spaces that are real and accessible to them. I see expert carework as an accessible way to reconfigure identities for caregivers, to think about differences anew, and to shape structures to better match their realities and meet their needs.

Paradox Two: The Duality of Lay/Expert Medical Agency and Control

Becoming an expert caregiver highlights a second interesting paradox associated with the medicalization of human conditions and behaviors. Existing research on the "double-edged sword of medicalization" (Riessman, 1983) and "ambivalent medicalization"

(Mauldin, 2016) highlights the tricky individual agency and structural control dynamics inherent in empirical cases of medicalization today. Specifically, throughout chapters 3 through 5, we see how, in the attempt to secure a diagnosis and subsequent services, enact policy reforms, challenge dominant lay/expert knowledge production, and increase public awareness of autism as a disability, not a disease, caregivers are simultaneously enabling and challenging medicalization. For example, caregivers appropriate expert knowledge as a means to minimize the power and knowledge distance between expert and nonexpert and gain entrée into previously off-limits professional and medical realms, while at the same time they defer to biomedical framings of autism to secure accommodations in school and insurance coverage of support interventions. By operating within the private sphere and through biomedical frameworks, autism remains individualized and medicalized.

Narratives articulate the importance of a formal medical diagnosis to qualify for life-altering services and insurance coverage, as well as to legitimize and understand caregivers' experiences. In doing so, they actively expand the jurisdiction of medicine to include individual family life and extramedical systems like education and social policy. Lay caregivers are implicated in the dominance of the medical approach to autism due to current structural arrangements that hamstring their ability to access necessary services, spaces, and legitimacy without a medical diagnosis. As Frank Furedi (2006) states, "the most significant developments that shape the process of contemporary medicalization are generated outside the institution of medicine" (p. 17).

On the other hand, expert caregiving can also function as a demedicalizing force by challenging the top-down expertise of medical professionals and formal institutions as the sole authority to frame autism and the caring experience. Demedicalizing practices extend legitimacy to understand and "treat" autism beyond the medical institution, and in this case, recognize caregivers' experiential knowledge and the need to take seriously nonmedical factors in autism discussions and interventions. More specifically, founding medical sociologist Renee Fox (1977) defines demedicalization as a "critical perspective that links the labeling of illness, the 'imperialist' outlook and capitalist behavior of physicians, the 'stigmatizing' and 'dehumanizing' experiences of patients, and the problems of the health-care system more generally to imperfections and injustices in the society as a whole" (p. 18). Such a transformation away from medical dominance and physician control allows an opportunity to shift the framing of autism from an individual medical problem to a broader social issue of disability. In other words, demedicalization can help to blur the medical gaze by affording nonmedical entities, like lay caregivers, agentic legitimacy in labeling and framing autism.

Caregiver agency and self-efficacy are developed through this process of challenging the supremacy of hierarchical and paternalistic institutions like medicine and health care. Evidence in this study shows how caregivers are active, agentic players in the co-construction of a medical diagnosis and therapeutic plan. They play a significant role in defining and framing their children's behaviors, which challenges the top-down power structure between healthcare provider and family caregiver. In most cases, caregivers take the helm in creating a therapeutic plan and securing support services. The everyday therapeutic support plan is driven, managed, and reformed by caregivers, who act as a mechanism to subvert the cultural authority of medicine and legitimize experiential knowledge. Therefore, this section highlights the paradoxical relationships among expert caregiving, medicalization, and demedicalization, which complicates the lived experiences of caregivers and their families. Further, the duality of medicalization significantly impacts autism carework, and caregivers continue to live in this amorphous space between often contradictory worlds.

The Power of Carework and Revealing Structural Flaws in "The Rest of the World"

Narratives that describe the process of becoming an expert caregiver reveal structural invisibilities and flaws at the levels of identity, institutions, and culture, and provide insight into ways to address these often forgotten yet critical aspects of the caring experience. Expert caregiving becomes a pragmatic way to reclaim power and assert one's agency in what feels like an out-of-control and structurally deterministic experience. The expert caregiver toolkit includes wide-ranging competencies that boost caregivers' sense of self-confidence and self-efficacy and allow them to shape mainstream institutional practices and naturalized discourses about autism through their everyday carework practices at grocery stores, at family holiday events, and in schools and doctors' offices. Expert caregiving produces tangible results that caregivers can see, hear, feel, and touch, and in doing so, reminds them, after years of waiting and frustrating institutional blocks, of their capacity to determine their own family's lives with significant identity impacts.

Specifically, expert caregiving becomes a means to reconfigure and repair ruptures in self-identity, negative emotional states, and especially feelings of isolation and marginalization. Through reflection, caregivers identify the social and personal drivers of their personal identity struggles and seek out ways to repair and heal, oftentimes through community. In doing so, carework activities become a ground to take care of their children and themselves.

Caregivers become diagnosticians, therapists, nutritionists, teachers, and advocates (and more) because of the systematic gaps that they experience firsthand throughout the diagnostic process, and later, in the everyday relational caring experience that involves multiple institutions. The road to the diagnosis is winding and bumpy, and expensive resources are cobbled together and hard to find because these systems are set up to be this way. The unsatisfying and isolating experiences that caregivers share reflect the ways that current social arrangements exclude the lived realities and needs of whole groups of people. Here, carework becomes a way to fill institutional holes and structural gaps in an overtaxed, fragmented healthcare system and an underresourced educational system, while also challenging ableist and sexist cultural norms.

Accordingly, expert caregiving spotlights the need for a number of institutional reforms in health care, education, and the formal paid workplace. For example, almost all caregivers noted the need for coordinated, full-scope health care and therapeutic support services for the child and whole family. Coordinated care means that all of a child's healthcare practitioners speak to one another, are in regular contact, and co-construct a holistic healthcare plan. Further, all these services, ideally, would be located physically in the same place to receive true wrap-around care in a convenient and accessible manner. These principles would be extended to family-centered and caregiver-centered care, as well. For example, tensions and identity ruptures especially at the beginning of caregiver autism journeys show that caregivers need access to a variety of support resources, such as mental health counseling, marriage counseling to help with marital tensions, quality babysitters or respite care experienced with neurodivergent children, and help with domestic labor.

Additionally, the incompatibility between the intensification of unpaid family carework and paid work outside of the home creates an often unacknowledged aspect in autism discussions. As Jane states, "I mean, people always forget about the job aspect. Every time I go somewhere you always hear about the medical stuff. . . . It's expensive to do this, expensive to do that. But you don't hear about how difficult it is to find a flexible job that understands our situation or to keep a job." A workplace culture that understands her situation is one that allows her to run to school if her son's teacher calls, or to adjust her schedule outside of the traditional workday to take her son to therapies. Many women were forced to leave their jobs because of inflexible workplace requirements that are structured on antiquated norms of separate spheres and do not allow them to meet vital caregiving needs. As Jane concludes, "I can't work a 9-to-5 every day with no flexibility. I'm damn good at my job and willing to take a pay cut for a company that just allows me to do my job, without making me physically be in the office all the time. There's no monetary value that you can place on stuff like that."

Similarly, the structure of many in-home autism services requires a caregiver to be home during regular work hours, which again reflects entrenched U.S. gendered norms of work and family.

As Adelina, mother of a three-year-old boy, states, "And that's the Catch-22: you can't work if you need to be at home, never mind being able to afford childcare. So therefore, if you can't pull in extra income, how do you pay the rent and just meet our basic needs? We're trying to figure out a way for me to stay home, but we're struggling financially." Therefore, caregiver narratives elucidate often invisible structural challenges, here in the realm of formal work, that are a part of the caring experience that deeply affect their everyday lives and promote inequalities.

However, the intensification of carework seen throughout this study is not just a result of institutional gaps and social marginalization. For some, it is also a purposeful strategy to shift the paradigm on autism away from pathological disorder to social disability and an appreciation for neurodiversity. For some caregivers, the values and goals that drive community carework include community building and amplifying the social model of autism. To a great degree, community carework activities involve a significant critique of the biomedical model's conceptualization of autism—the conventional science on etiology, diagnostic process, and primary treatment methods. Accordingly, narratives in this book show how everyday forms of expert caregiving can be a mechanism to shape understandings of autism and disability, gender and family, and formal institutions like education and health care. The expert caregiver emerges as a space to repair ruptures in identity, democratize access to resources and knowledge, build community and social inclusion, and engage in collective action aimed at structural changes, all within a constrained and contested landscape.

Over and over again, I hear stories of families struggling with the same issues and waging the same battles—how to be referred for an autism evaluation, how to secure therapeutic services, what accommodations are available to ask for in IEP meetings, and more. Therefore, the pervasive and uncertain nature of the autism caring experience demonstrates the effects of infrastructure gaps and social processes of ableism on everyday life, and the shifting of responsibility from professionals, policy, and institutions onto individual caregivers. The narratives in this book help to shift our focus onto the flaws in surrounding care systems and entrenched cultural expectations that make the social caring experience so arduous for mothers.

Carework is disproportionately done by women across the globe, overwhelmingly unpaid, underacknowledged, and rendered invisible. This is a story that I hope sheds broader light on how structural flaws intensify and complicate essential carework for a growing number of young families caring for neurodivergent, disabled, medically fragile, and/or chronically ill children. Following the feminist ethic of care, I intend for this book to help prioritize attention to the complexities of carework and to elevate the status of caregivers in our society.

Appendix A
Methodology and Caregiver Demographics

My research questions necessitate the use of qualitative research methods in the form of individual intensive informal interviews and participant-observation fieldwork to understand the lived experiences and meaning-making processes for primary caregivers of autistic and neurodivergent children under the age of 18 years. My research includes over two years of participant-observation at two primary sites that are autism parent and caregiver support group meetings, both located in Northern California.

For both groups, the meetings are semistructured with a moderator, and the agendas vary monthly. Sometimes, there are specific topics or presentations around which the meetings are organized. Other times, there is a longer question-and-answer or open discussion period. Groups meet monthly for two hours and are attended by, on average, thirty primary caregivers, most of whom are women between the ages of thirty and fifty-five, and most of whom are mothers of an autistic child. I found all organizations and meetings through a web search of local autism groups and contacted the program managers to set up introductory meetings and to join their email listservs. I also attended and observed a variety of onetime community resource and informational meetings, autism research talks, and educational community events.

In the tradition of fieldwork and grounded theory (Glaser & Strauss, 1967), this study is based on observation and in-depth interviews with mothers and is centered physically and theoretically within the home and family, where I spent on average 2.5 hours in the privacy of their homes, while discussing their lives and experiences as primary caregivers. Interviews ranged from two to four hours' total in length and were audio recorded and later transcribed verbatim. During interviews, siblings were often playing in the background, or our conversation would be paused in order for the caregiver to attend to a crying infant or to take a call from a babysitter currently watching her children. Frequently, I was asked to hold a baby while a mom tended to her other child or put on the kettle for tea or simply took a moment to wipe away tears. I met the caregivers' children, they invited me into the safety and privacy of their homes and worlds, and their guards were down. I was continually taken aback by the honesty, purpose, and ease with which each caregiver spoke in telling me about her family's experiences. It was made abundantly clear to me that these mothers needed to tell their stories, and they absolutely needed to be heard.

I began each interview by discussing my genuine interest in the complexities associated with autism and caregiving concerns for families with autistic children. Some mothers jumped in right away and started the conversation. With more reticent respondents, I began by asking them to tell me about their family. Our conversations then addressed a series of topics, largely dependent on the child's age and life experiences. Such topics include how the diagnosis was received, typical everyday family life (sibling relationships, marriages, extended family relationships), experiences in schools and with the educational system, healthcare experiences with medical professionals, current therapeutic team and experiences with diverse interventions, and fears and hopes for the future.

Appendix B features the interview schedule that roughly guided each conversation, though I always let the women lead the conversation. I allowed participants to guide our conversations, skip anything too triggering, and focus discussion on areas that were of most importance and salient to them personally.

Many of my interviews involved heavy emotional sharing and discussion of heart-wrenching life experiences. For example, a mother told me how she slept on the floor next to her child's bed for six months because he was suicidal from years of bullying in school, and she was afraid he was going to self-harm. The openness and extent to which women were able and willing to share their stories and hardships were remarkable. I feel this speaks very loudly to the silence and lack of support and understanding felt within the broader autism community by the public. Many parents just want to be heard and to have their experiences validated, and I feel honored to voice these stories.

In total, I conducted fifty in-depth semistructured interviews with mothers of at least one child under the age of eighteen years with an official autism diagnosis. All eligible interviewees had to be the primary caregiver of a dependent child who was under eighteen years old, diagnosed with autism, autism spectrum disorder, or Asperger's syndrome, and lived in Northern California to meet face-to-face for an interview. It is important to note that my entire sample includes children whose primary diagnosis would now fit under the autism spectrum disorder diagnosis, according to the latest *DSM-V* manual (APA, 2022). All children ranged in age from five years to seventeen years, though the median age was ten years old. An overwhelming majority of the children in this sample were under twelve years old and male. Of the total fifty interviews, only 20 percent of mothers had daughters diagnosed with autism; the remaining 80 percent had sons with autism, which is representative of the disproportionate diagnosis for boys. Nationally, autism has been four times more common in boys than girls, though the gender gap is beginning to decrease (CDC, 2023). For the first time, the CDC (2023) has reported that the prevalence of autism among eight-year-old girls has exceeded 1 percent. Additionally, 12 percent of the total families had more than one child diagnosed with autism, and four of the children in this study were adopted.

All interviewee participants ranged in age from twenty-eight to fifty years, with a mean age of thirty-seven years. A disproportionate number of mothers had a higher education, for example, twenty-seven women held a bachelor's degree, and nine held master's degrees. The overwhelming majority of interviewees are married (forty-eight married, and two divorced) and self-identify as middle-class. Of the forty-eight married women, their husbands all worked full-time outside the home. Of the women interviewed, twenty-two were full-time stay-at-home mothers, thirteen worked part-time jobs outside the home, and thirteen worked full-time jobs outside the home. Self-identification of race or ethnicity of caregivers is as follows: 70 percent White, 12 percent Latina, 8 percent Asian, 10 percent Mixed Race. For more detailed demographic information on the sample, please see the following Table A.1. This sample is disproportionately white, college educated, and middle class, with an autistic son, which matches dominant autism demographics. However, autism is prevalent in children of all races, genders, and socioeconomic classes, and girls with autism are often underdiagnosed or misdiagnosed.

All interview participants were recruited via convenience and snowball sampling, after receiving Institutional Review Board (IRB) approval. I advertised widely for study participants in various mothers of autistic children "Meet-Up" groups, in a social networking site, and in local autism clinics and social skills groups, as well as in public spaces, such as local coffee shops and public libraries. All interviews were set up via email, in which I introduced myself and the focus of this study. After initial interviews with mothers, I often received additional interviewees through word of mouth to their peers and other mothers with children with autism. The majority of interviews were conducted in mothers' homes throughout Northern California, and the minority were conducted in local public places, such as a coffee shop, a public library, or a mother's work office space.

I employed a variety of analysis techniques throughout the data collection process. For each field site visit, I would take copious notes by hand, paying attention to individual actions and behaviors (including tone, nonverbal gestures, and facial expressions) and group social interaction (i.e., who is interacting with whom and how?). I also paid special attention to the types of questions asked and the form of the answers given in the field resource meetings.

TABLE A.1 Caregiver Demographics (all self-reported data)

NAME	AGE	MARITAL STATUS	RACE/ ETHNICITY	OCCUPATION	HIGHEST LEVEL OF EDUCATION	SOCIAL CLASS
Sarah	35	Married	White	Mother	BA	Middle class
Laurie	45	Married	White	Financial analyst	MA	Middle class
Brynn	32	Married	White	Office manager	BA	Middle class
Danielle	31	Married	White	Mother	AA	Middle class
Katie	38	Married	White	Realtor*	BA	Middle class
Anne	42	Married	White	Event planner	BA	Middle class
Catherine	45	Married	Asian	Mother	BA	Middle class
Debbie	36	Married	Latina	Mother	HS	Middle class
Stephanie	30	Married	Asian & White	Mother	BA	Middle class
Jennifer	34	Married	African American & White	Mother	HS	Middle class
Maria	35	Married	Latina	Mother	BA	Middle class
Candace	41	Married	White	Therapist*	MA	Middle class
Rebecca	35	Married	Asian & White	Marketing	MA	Middle class
Mallory	37	Divorced	White	Office assistant	AA	Middle class
Jane	50	Married	White	CPA	MA	Middle class
Maya	44	Married	White	Realtor	BA	Middle class
Liz	31	Married	Latina & White	Mother	BA	Middle class
Marianne	36	Divorced	White	Medical billing*	AA	Middle class
Amy	46	Married	Latina & African American	Mother	HS	Middle class

(*Continued*)

TABLE A.1 (*Continued*)

NAME	AGE	MARITAL STATUS	RACE/ ETHNICITY	OCCUPATION	HIGHEST LEVEL OF EDUCATION	SOCIAL CLASS
Stacey	38	Married	White	Retail*	HS	Middle class
Lisa	36	Married	White	Graphic designer	BA	Middle class
Serena	33	Married	Latina	Mother	HS	Middle class
Kristen	39	Married	White	Office admin*	BA	Middle class
Leah	42	Married	White	Office admin*	BA	Middle class
Joanne	29	Married	White	Mother	BA	Working Class
Claire	37	Married	White	Preschool teacher*	BA	Middle class
Colleen	40	Married	White	Mother	HS	Middle class
Mary	48	Married	Latina	Project manager	BA	Middle class
Susan	33	Married	White	Admin asst*	MA	Middle class
Beth	36	Married	White	Mother	AA	Middle class
Aimee	39	Married	White	Daycare teacher*	AA	Middle class
Emma	30	Married	Asian	Mother	BA	Middle class
Anna	32	Married	White	IT specialist	MA	Middle class
Carole	36	Married	Asian	Mother	BA	Middle class
Dana	31	Married	White	Web design*	MA	Middle class
Samantha	34	Married	White	Mother	BA	Middle class
Alexandra	32	Married	White	Mother	BA	Middle class
Yvette	35	Married	White	Counselor*	MA	Middle class
Kendra	43	Married	White	Mother	HS	Middle class

TABLE A.1 (*Continued*)

NAME	AGE	MARITAL STATUS	RACE/ ETHNICITY	OCCUPATION	HIGHEST LEVEL OF EDUCATION	SOCIAL CLASS
Leah	42	Married	White	Admin asst*	BA	Middle class
Shelly	37	Married	White	CPA*	BA	Middle class
Karen	28	Married	Asian	HR manager	BA	Middle class
Brenna	35	Married	White	Mother	BA	Middle class
Rachel	37	Married	Latina	Office admin	AA	Middle class
Fiona	38	Married	White	Mother	AA	Middle class
Adelina	42	Married	Latina	Librarian*	MA	Middle class
Terri	39	Married	White	Counselor*	BA	Middle class
Isabel	34	Married	White	Mother	BA	Middle class
Lizzy	36	Married	White	Mother	BA	Middle class
Charlotte	43	Married	White	Marketing	BA	Middle class

NOTES: *= Part-time employment. All names included in this table are pseudonyms.

Immediately after each field visit and interview, I would spend about one hour processing the event, by jotting down notes by hand on the major themes and key quotations raised in the interview. Then, I would formalize and extend these notes into a typed short "memo" (Lofland et al., 2011; Emerson, 1995) to begin making sense of the data and connecting them to theoretical ideas. After all interviews were transcribed, this study used thematic analysis (Braun & Clarke, 2006) to code the data in multiple stages. Following the principle of "repeated reading" (Braun & Clarke, 2006), I reread the transcripts and field notes multiple times to identify themes in the data and then hone into codes and subcodes.

I further organized and clarified the data into key codes and analytic themes during the earliest stages of the writing process.

Methodological Implications and Limits

I purposefully privilege the stories and voices of mothers who often were systematically and formally silenced throughout their early autism journeys, and who continue to "fight" and struggle for cultural legitimacy—simply, to be heard and valued. To do so, my data collection was largely sited in the private realm—on the couch in the family room, or at the kitchen table within each individual family's home. Accordingly, the interview schedule was guided by participants, and in this way, I was able to receive incredibly intimate, authentic, and unfiltered narratives of their lives.

Therefore, this study design offers an authentic interpretation of the social experience of autism caregiving particularly from the ground up. However, the design of the study has some weaknesses. Primarily, it features only one side of the autism caring story: lay caregivers, who are 100 percent women and predominately mothers in this study. Thus, it ignores the different perspectives within the family, from partners, grandparents, and siblings, as well as professional and medical insight. My data do not include any interviews with medical professionals or specialists, nor did I conduct any fieldwork within the formal clinical context. My findings could be strengthened and made more generalizable if I included the words and experiences of autism medical experts and specialists, as well as insight from additional lay family members (fathers and siblings, in particular). In most families with more than one child, often mothers would express concerns associated with sibling relationships. Therefore, future research could center on neurodiverse sibling relationships and the intensification of carework from siblings' perspectives. The constrained picture of the autism caring experience needs to be noted for methodological and theoretical implications.

Appendix B
Interview Schedule

1. Please tell me about yourself, your family, and your child (ren).
2. Please tell me about the first few years of your child's development. Did you have any concerns?
3. How did the early well-baby checks (the first visits) with your pediatrician go? What did they recommend? How did you feel when leaving these visits?
4. Please describe the diagnostic process. Did you experience any obstacles, problems, or roadblocks in getting your child diagnosed and treated? Who/what do you consider the most valuable resources that aided you in the diagnostic process?
5. Please describe a typical day in your life and household. What do you consider a good day and a challenging one, and why?
6. How do you define and understand autism? "Wat does it mean to you?
7. What are the most important resources and sources of help in your life right now? What services, experts, any forms of support and assistance for your child do you receive outside of your pediatrician and family? What is lacking? Does your insurance cover most of the services you have?
8. Please tell me about your engagement in the community.
9. Please tell me about your experiences with schools, teachers, and administrators. Are there things that the educational system does not provide that you need, or that you have sought elsewhere?

10. In terms of support services and resources for you and your family, what do you need/want? What do you wish you had, in terms of support services for you, your child, and family as a whole?
11. What advice do you have for others negotiating and navigating the educational system and medical system, etc.?
12. For parents who are just beginning their autism journeys, what would you like to say to them? Do you have anything else you would like to share?

Acknowledgments

I would like to express my sincere gratitude to a number of people who have helped me to complete this book. This book is the culmination of the intellectual guidance and encouragement provided by Ming-Cheng Lo, Diane Wolf, Michael McQuarrie, and Debora Paterniti in my academic training as a sociologist at the University of California, Davis. I am grateful for all your support in fostering my skills, growth, and sociological interests as a scholar. This book has come to fruition with the support of Mignon Duffy, Amy Armenia, and Kim Price-Glynn and the editorial team at Rutgers University Press. Thank you and an anonymous reviewer for the rounds of thoughtful constructive feedback and for seeing the potential of this project to make a meaningful contribution to care scholarship.

There would be no book without the willingness of fifty caregivers to share their stories with open hearts. I am grateful for the honesty and courage with which these women told their stories, and for trusting me to voice them accurately.

It is only with the unwavering love and support of my family and cherished friends that I was able to complete this book. I am heavily indebted to my parents, Claudia and Alan, my husband Benjamin, Laura Fineman's editing eye, and dear friends Shelly Buchanan-Cello, Laurie Shlala, Serenity Pang-Bellman, Brad DeMont, and Setarreh Massihzadegan who have helped cheer me and this project along especially in moments of doubt. Thank you.

References

Abel, E. K., & Nelson, M. K. (1990). Circles of care: An introductory essay. In E. K. Abel and M. K. Nelson (Eds.), *Circles of care: Work and identity in women's lives* (pp. 105–131). Albany: State University of New York Press.

Allen, K. R., & Walker, A. J. (1992). Attentive love: A feminist perspective on the caregiving of adult daughters. *Family Relations, 41*(3), 284–289.

American Psychiatric Association (APA). (1952). *Diagnostic and statistical manual of mental disorders.*

———. (1980). *Diagnostic and statistical manual of mental disorders* (3rd ed.).

———. (1994). *Diagnostic and statistical manual of mental disorders* (4th ed.).

———. (2013). *Diagnostic and statistical manual of mental disorders* (5th ed.).

———. (2022). *Diagnostic and statistical manual of mental disorders* (5th ed., text rev.).

Anderson, L. K. (2023). Autistic experiences of applied behavior analysis. *Autism, 27*(3), 737–750.

Armenia, A. B. (2009). More than motherhood: Reasons for becoming a family day care provider. *Journal of Family Issues, 30*(4), 554–574.

Asperger, H. (1944). Die Autistiesehen Psychopathen in Kindesalter. *Arch. Psych. Nervenkrankh, 117*, 76–136.

Barker, K. K. (2005). *The fibromyalgia story: Medical authority and women's worlds of pain.* Philadelphia: Temple University Press.

———. (2008). Electronic support groups, patient-consumers, and medicalization: The case of contested illness. *Journal of Health and Social Behavior, 49*, 20–36.

Bettelheim, B. (1967). *The empty fortress: Infantile autism and the birth of the self.* New York: Free Press.

Bleuler, E. (1911 [1950]). *Dementia praecox or the group of schizophrenias.* Oxford: International Universities Press.

Blum, L. M. (2007). Mother-blame in the Prozac Nation: Raising kids with invisible disabilities. *Gender & Society, 21,* 202–226.

———. (2015). *Raising Generation Rx: Mothering kids with invisible disabilities in an age of inequality.* New York: New York University Press.

Bourdieu, P. (1979). *La Distinction.* Paris: Editions de Minuit.

Braun, V., & Clarke, V. (2006). Using thematic analysis in psychology. *Qualitative Research in Psychology, 3*(2), 77–101.

Brenton, J. (2017). The limits of intensive feeding: Maternal foodwork at the intersections of race, class, and gender. *Sociology of Health & Illness, 39*(6), 863–877.

Brown, P. (1992). Popular epidemiology and toxic waste contamination: Lay and professional ways of knowing. *Journal of Health and Social Behavior, 33*(3), 267–281.

Budig, M. J., & Misra, J. (2010). How care-work employment shapes earnings in cross-national perspective. *International Labour Review, 149,* 441–460.

Bury, M. (2000). On chronic illness and disability. In C. Bird, P. Conrad, and A. M. Fremont (Eds.), *Handbook of medical sociology* (pp. 173–183). Upper Saddle River, NJ: Prentice Hall.

Cancian, F. M., & Oliker, S. J. (2000). *Caring and gender.* Thousand Oaks, CA: Pine Forge Press.

Carey, A. C., Block, P., & Scotch, R. (2020). *Allies and obstacles: Disability activism and parents of children with disabilities.* Philadelphia: Temple University Press.

Carr, E. G. (1977). The motivation of self-injurious behavior: A review of some hypotheses. *Psychological Bulletin, 84*(4), 800.

Centers for Disease Control and Prevention (CDC). (2023). Autism Spectrum Disorders (ASDs): Data and statistics. http://www.cdc.gov/ncbddd/autism/data.htm

Charmaz, K. (2000). Experiencing chronic illness. In G. L. Albrecht, R. Fitzpatrick, and S. Scrimshaw (Eds.), *Handbook of social studies in health and medicine* (pp. 277–292). London: Sage Publications.

———. (2020). Experiencing stigma and exclusion: The influence of neoliberal perspectives, practices, and policies on living with chronic illness and disability. *Symbolic Interaction, 43*(1), 21–45.

Chiaraluce, C. A. (2018). Narratives on the autism journey: "Doing family" and redefining the caregiver self. *Journal of Family Issues, 39*(10), 2883–2905.

Chodorow, N. J. (1978). *The reproduction of mothering: Psychoanalysis and the sociology of gender*. Los Angeles: University of California Press.

Christopher, K. (2012). Extensive mothering: Employed mothers' constructions of the good mother. *Gender and Society, 26*(1), 73–96.

Cohen, H., Amerine-Dickens, M., & Smith, T. (2006). Early intensive behavioral treatment: Replication of the UCLA Model in a community setting. *Journal of Developmental and Behavioral Pediatrics, 27*, 5145–5155.

Conrad, P. (1992). Medicalization and social control. *Annual Review of Sociology, 18*, 209–232.

———. (2007). *The medicalization of society: On the transformation of human conditions into treatable disorders*. Baltimore: Johns Hopkins University Press.

Corburn, J. (2005). *Street science: Community knowledge and environmental health justice*. Cambridge, MA: MIT Press.

Davidson, G., Smith, D., & Frankel, S. (1991). Lay epidemiology and the prevention paradox: The implications of coronary candidacy for health education. *Sociology of Health & Illness, 13*(1), 1–19.

Davies, C. (1995). Competence versus care? Gender and caring work revisited. *Acta Sociologica, 38*, 17–31.

DeMyer, M. K., Hingtgen, J. N., & Jackson, R. K. (1981). Infantile autism reviewed: A decade of research. *Schizophrenia Bulletin, 7*(3), 388–451.

DeVault, M. L. (1991). *Feeding the family: The social organization of caring as gendered work*. Chicago: University of Chicago Press.

Dow, D. M. (2019). *Mothering while Black: Boundaries and burdens of middle-class parenthood*. Oakland: University of California Press.

Duffy, M. (2011). *Making care count: A century of gender, race, and paid care work*. New Brunswick, NJ: Rutgers University Press.

Duffy, M., Armenia, A., & Stacey, C. (2015). *Caring on the clock: The complexities and contradictions of paid care work*. New Brunswick, NJ: Rutgers University Press.

Eikeseth, S. (2009). Outcome of comprehensive psycho-educational interventions for young children with autism. *Research in Developmental Disabilities, 30*, 158–178.

Eisenberg, N., & Mussen, P. H. (1989). *The roots of prosocial behavior in children*. New York: Wiley.

Eldevik S., Eikeseth, S., Jahr, E., & Smith, T. (2006). Effects of low-intensity behavioral treatment for children with autism and mental retardation. *Journal of Autism and Developmental Disorders, 36*, 211–224.

Eldevik S., Hastings, R. P., Jahr, E., & Hughes, J. C. (2012). Outcomes of behavioral intervention for children with autism in mainstream pre-school settings. *Journal of Autism and Developmental Disorders, 42*(2), 210–220.

Emerson, R. M., Fretz, R. I., & Shaw, L. L. (1995). *Writing ethnographic fieldnotes*. Chicago: University of Chicago Press.

Engels, F. ([1884] 1972). *The origins of the family, private property, and the state*. New York: International Publishers.

England, P. (1992). *Comparable worth: Theories and evidence*. New York: Aldine DeGruyter.

———. (2005). Emerging theories of care work. *Annual Review of Sociology, 31*(1), 381–399.

England, P., Budig, M., & Folbre, N. (2002). Wages of virtue: Relative pay of care work. *Social Problems, 49*, 455–473.

Ezzy, D. (2000). Illness narratives: Time, hope and HIV. *Social Science & Medicine, 50*, 605–617.

Finkelstein, V. (2001a). A personal journey into disability politics. *The Disability Studies Archive UK*, Center for Disability Studies, University of Leeds.

———. (2001b). The social model repossessed. *The Disability Studies Archive UK*, Center for Disability Studies, University of Leeds.

Folbre, N. (2001). *The invisible heart: Economics and family values*. New York: New Press.

Fox, R. C. (1977). The medicalization and demedicalization of American society. *Daedalus*, Winter, 9–22.

Frank, A. (1995). *The wounded storyteller: Body, illness, and ethics*. Chicago: University of Chicago Press.

Freitag, C. M. (2007). The genetics of autistic disorders and its clinical relevance: A review of the literature. *Molecular Psychiatry, 12*(1), 2–22.

Furedi, F. (2006). The end of professional dominance. *Society, 43*, 14–18.

Geschwind, D. H. (2009). Advances in autism. *Annual Review of Medicine, 60*, 367–380.

Gibson, J. L., Pritchard, E., & de Lemos, C. (2021). Play-based interventions to support social and communication development in autistic children aged 2–8 years: A scoping review. *Autism & Developmental Language Impairments, 6*, 1–30.

Gibson, M. F., & Douglas, P. (2018). Disturbing behaviors: Ole Ivar Lovaas and the queer history of autism science. *Catalyst: Feminism, Theory, Technoscience, 4*(2), 1–28.

Glaser, B. G., & Strauss, A. L. (1967). *The discovery of grounded theory: Strategies for qualitative research.* Hawthorne, NY: Aldine de Gruyter.

Glenn, E. N. (1992). From servitude to service work: Historical continuities in the racial division of paid reproductive labor. *Signs: Journal of Women in Culture and Society, 18*, 1–43.

Good, B. (1994). *Medicine, rationality and experience.* Cambridge: Cambridge University Press.

Good, M. J. (2007). The biotechnical embrace and the medical imaginary. In J. Biehl, B. Good, and A. Kleinman (Eds.), *Subjectivity: Ethnographic investigations* (pp. 362–380). Berkeley: University of California Press.

Good, M.J.D., & Good, B. (2000). Clinical narratives and the study of contemporary doctor-patient relationships. In G. L. Albrecht, R. Fitzpatrick, and S. Scrimshaw (Eds.), *Handbook of social studies in health and medicine* (pp. 243–258). Thousand Oaks, CA: SAGE.

Gordon, S., Benner, P., & Noddings, N. (1996). *Caregiving: Readings in knowledge, practice, ethics and politics.* Philadelphia: University of Pennsylvania Press.

Gordon-Lipkin, E., Foster, J., & Peacock, G. (2016). Whittling down the wait time: Exploring models to minimize the delay from initial concern to diagnosis and treatment of autism spectrum disorder. *Pediatric Clinics of North America, 63*(5), 851–859.

Grandin, T., & Panek, R. (2013). *The autistic brain: Thinking across the spectrum.* Boston: Houghton Mifflin Harcourt.

Gray, D. E. (1993). Perceptions of stigma: The parents of autistic children. *Sociology of Health and Illness, 15*(1), 102–120.

———. (2001). Accommodation, resistance and transcendence: Three narratives of autism. *Social Science & Medicine, 53*, 1247–1257.

———. (2002). "Everybody just freezes. Everybody is just embarrassed": Felt and enacted stigma among parents of children with high functioning autism. *Sociology of Health and Illness, 24*, 734–749.

———. (2003). Gender and coping: The parents of children with high functioning autism. *Social Science & Medicine, 56*(3), 631–642.

Green, S. E. (2007). "We're tired, not sad": Benefits and burdens of mothering a child with a disability. *Social Science & Medicine, 64*(1), 150–163.

Ha, S., Sohn, I., Kim, N., Sim, H. J., & Cheon, K. A. (2015). Characteristics of brains in autism spectrum disorder: Structure, function and connectivity across the lifespan. *Experimental Neurobiology, 24*(4), 273–284.

Happé, F., & Frith, U. (2020). Annual research review: Looking back to look forward—changes in the concept of autism and implications for future research. *Journal of Child Psychology and Psychiatry, 61*, 218–232.

Happé, F., Ronald, A., & Plomin, R. (2006). Time to give up on a single explanation for autism. *Nature Neuroscience, 9*(10), 1218–1220.

Hays, S. (1996). *The cultural contradictions of motherhood*. New Haven, CT: Yale University Press.

Herbert, M. R. (2010). Contributions of the environment and environmentally vulnerable physiology to autism spectrum disorders. *Current Opinion in Neurology, 23*(2), 103–110.

Herbert, M. R., Russo, J. P., Yang, S., Roohi, J., Blaxill, M., Kahler, S. G., Cremer, L., & Hatchwell, E. (2006). Autism and environmental genomics. *NeuroToxicology, 27*, 671–684.

Herd, P., & Meyer, M. H. (2002). Care work: Invisible civic engagement. *Gender & Society, 16*(5), 665–688.

Hochschild, A. (1983). *The managed heart: Commercialization of human feeling*. Berkeley: University of California Press.

———. (1995). The culture of politics: Traditional, postmodern, cold-modern, and warm-modern ideals of care. *Social Politics, 2*(3), 331–346.

Hughes, J. M. (2016). *Increasing neurodiversity in disability and social justice advocacy groups*. White paper. Autistic Self Advocacy Network. Available online at: https://autisticadvocacy.org/wp-content/uploads/2016/06/whitepaper-Increasing-Neurodiversity-in-Disability-and-Social-Justice-Advocacy-Groups.pdf (accessed March 1, 2023).

Institute of Medicine. (2004). Health literacy: A prescription to end confusion. *National Academy of Sciences*, April 8.

Jarrett, R. L., & Jefferson, S. R. (2003). "A good mother got to fight for her kids": Maternal management strategies in a high-risk, African-American neighborhood. *Journal of Children and Poverty, 9*, 21–39.

Johnson, C. P., & Myers, S. M. (2007). American Academy of Pediatrics Council on Children with Disabilities Identification and evaluation of children with autism spectrum disorders. *Pediatrics, 120*(5), 1183–1215.

Kanner, L. (1943). Autistic disturbances of affective contact. *Nervous Child, 2*, 217–250.

———. (1949). Problems of nosology and psychodynamics of early infantile autism. *American Journal of Orthopsychiatry, 19*(3), 416–426.

Kibria, K., & Suarez Becerra, W. (2021). Deserving immigrants and good advocate mothers: Immigrant mothers' negotiations of special education systems for children with disabilities. *Social Problems, 68*(3), 591–607.

Kleinman, A. (1988). *The illness narratives: Suffering, healing, and the human condition*. New York: Basic Books.

Landsman, G. H. (1998). Reconstructing motherhood in the age of "perfect" babies: Mothers of infants and toddlers with disabilities. *Signs, 24*(1), 69–99.

———. (2008). *Reconstructing motherhood in the age of perfect babies*. New York: Routledge.

Lareau, A. (2011). *Unequal childhoods: Race, class, and family life*. Berkeley: University of California Press.

———. (2015). Cultural knowledge and social inequality. *American Sociological Review, 80*(1), 1–27.

Litt, J. (2004). Women's carework in low-income households: The special case of children with attention deficit hyperactivity disorder. *Gender & Society, 18*, 625–644.

Lofland, J., Snow, D., Anderson, L., & Lofland, L. (2011). *Analyzing social settings: A guide to qualitative observation and analysis*. Belmont, CA: Wadsworth/Thomson Learning.

Lovaas, O. I. (1987). Behavioral treatment and normal educational and intellectual functioning in young autistic children. *Journal of Consulting and Clinical Psychology, 55*(1), 3–9.

Lovaas, O. I., Berberich, J. P., Perloff, B. F., & Schaeffer, B. (1966). Acquisition of imitative speech by schizophrenic children. *Science, 151*, 705–707.

Lovaas, O., Schaeffer, B., & Simmons, J. (1965). Building social behavior in autistic children by use of electric shock. *Journal of Experimental Research in Personality, 1*, 99–109.

Maenner, M. J., Warren, Z., Williams, A. R., Amoakohene, E., Bakian, A. V., Bilder, D. A., Durkin, M. S., Fitzgerald, R. T., Furnier, S. M., Hughes, M. M., Ladd-Acosta, C. M., McArthur, D., Pas, E. T., Salinas, A., Vehorn, A., Williams, S., Esler, A., Grzybowski, A., Hall-Lande, J., Nguyen, R.H.N., Pierce, K., Zahorodny, W., Hudson, A., Hallas, L., Mancilla, K. C., Patrick, M., Shenouda, J., Sidwell, K., DiRienzo, M., Gutierrez, J., Spivey, M. H., Lopez, M., Pettygrove, S., Schwenk, Y. D., Washington, A., Shaw, K.A. (2023). "Prevalence and characteristics of autism spectrum disorder among children aged 8 years—Autism and developmental disabilities monitoring network, 11 sites, United States, 2020." *Morbidity and Mortality Weekly Report, 72*(2), 1–14.

Malacrida, C. (2003). *Cold comfort: Mothers, professionals, and attention deficit disorder.* Toronto: University of Toronto Press.

———. (2004). Medicalization, ambivalence and social control: Mothers' description of educators and ADD/ADHD. *Health: An Interdisciplinary Journal for the Social Study of Health, Illness and Medicine, 8*(1), 61–80.

Mattingly, C. (1994). The concept of therapeutic "emplotment." *Social Science and Medicine, 38*(6), 811–822.

———. (2012). *Paradox of hope: Journeys through a clinical borderland.* Berkeley: University of California Press.

Mattingly, C., & Garro, L. C. (2000). *Narrative and the cultural construction of illness and healing.* Berkeley: University of California Press.

Mauldin, L. (2016). *Made to hear: Cochlear implants and raising deaf children.* Minneapolis: University of Minnesota Press.

McEachin, J. J., Smith, T., & Lovaas, O. I. (1993). Long-term outcome for children with autism who received early intensive behavioral treatment. *American Journal on Mental Retardation, 97*(4), 359–372.

McGill, O., & Robinson, A. (2021). "Recalling hidden harms": Autistic experiences of childhood applied behavioural analysis (ABA). *Advances in Autism, 7*(4), 269–282.

McGuire, A. (2016). *War on autism: On the cultural logic of normative violence.* Ann Arbor: University of Michigan Press.

Miller, A. L., & Bogida, E. (2016). The Separate Spheres Model of gendered inequality. *PLoS One, 11*(1), 1–34.

Minshawi, N. F., Hurwitz, S., Fodstad, J. C., Biebl, S., Morriss, D. H., & McDougle, C. J. (2014). The association between self-injurious behaviors and autism spectrum disorders. *Psychology Research and Behavior Management, 7,* 125.

Mishler, E. (1984). *The discourse of medicine: Dialectics of medical interviews.* Norwood, NJ: Ablex.

———. (2005). Patient stories, narratives of resistance and the ethics of humane care. *Health, 9*(4), 431–451.

Misra, J. (2003). Caring about care. *Feminist Studies, 29,* 387–401.

Molloy, H., & Vasil, L. (2002). The social construction of Asperger syndrome: Pathologising difference. *Disability and Society, 17*(6), 659–669.

Oliver, M. (1990). *The politics of disablement.* London: Palgrave Macmillan.

———. (2013). The social model of disability: Thirty years on. *Disability & Society, 28*(7), 1024–1026.

Parks, J. A. (2003). *No place like home? Feminist ethics and home health care.* Bloomington: Indiana University Press.

Persico, A. M., & Bourgeron, T. (2006). Searching for ways out of the autism maze: Genetic, epigenetic and environmental clues. *Trends in Neuroscience, 29*(7), 349–358.

Reichow, B., Hume, K., Barton, E. E., & Boyd, B. A. (2018). Early intensive behavioral intervention (EIBI) for young children with autism spectrum disorders (ASD). *The Cochrane Database of Systematic Reviews, 5*(5), 009260.

Riessman, C. K. (1983). Women and medicalization: A new perspective. *Social Policy, 14*(1), 3–18.

Rogers, S. J., & Vismara, L. A. (2008). Evidence-based comprehensive treatments for early autism. *Journal of Clinical Child Adolescent Psychology, 37*(1), 8–38.

Sallows, G. O., & Graupner, T. D. (2005). Intensive behavioral treatment for children with autism: Four-year outcome and predictors. *American Journal of Mental Retardation, 6,* 417–438.

Schwartz, M., & Stryker, S. (1970). *Deviance, selves and others.* Washington, DC: American Sociological Association.

Shakespeare, T., & Watson, N. (2001). The social model of disability: An outdated ideology? In S. N. Barnartt and B. M. Altman (Eds.), *Exploring theories and expanding methodologies: Where we are and where we need to go* (Research in Social Science and Disability, Vol. 2) (pp. 9–28). Leeds: Emerald Group.

Silberman, S. (2015) *Neurotribes: The legacy of autism and the future of neurodiversity*. New York: Avery.

Singer, J. (1998). Odd people in: The birth of community amongst people on the "autistic spectrum": A personal exploration of a new social movement based on neurological diversity. Honours thesis, University of Technology, Sydney.

———. (1999). Why can't you be normal for once in your life?: From a "problem with no name" to a new category of disability. In M. Corker and S. French (Eds.), *Disability discourse* (pp. 59–67). Buckingham: Open University Press.

———. (2016). *NeuroDiversity: The birth of an idea*.

Singh, I. (2004). Doing their jobs: Mothering with Ritalin in a culture of mother-blame. *Social Science & Medicine, 59*, 1193–1205.

Singh, J. S. (2016). *Multiple autisms: Spectrums of advocacy and genomic science*. Minneapolis: University of Minnesota Press.

Smith, D., & Griffith, A. (1990). Coordinating the uncoordinated: Mothering, schooling, and the family wage. *Perspectives on Social Problems, 2*(1), 25–43.

Smith, D. E. (1993). The Standard North American Family: SNAF as an ideological code. *Journal of Family Issues, 14*(1), 50–65.

Smith, L. (n.d.). *Center for Disability Rights*. #Ableism—Center for Disability Rights. https://cdrnys.org/blog/uncategorized/ableism/

Somers, M. (1994). The narrative constitution of identity: A relational and network approach. *Theory and Society, 23*, 605–649.

Stenning, A., & Bertilsdotter-Rosqvist, H. (2021). Neurodiversity studies: Mapping out possibilities of a new critical paradigm. *Disability & Society, 36*(9), 1532–1537.

Tanner, D. (1999). The narrative imperative: Stories in medicine, illness and bioethics. *HEC Forum, 11*(2), 155–169.

Terrizzi, J., & Shook, N. (2020). On the origin of shame: Does shame emerge from an evolved disease-avoidance architecture? *Frontiers in Behavioral Neuroscience, 14*(19), 1–13.

Thomas, C. (2004a). How is disability understood? An examination of sociological approaches. *Disability & Society, 19*(6), 569–583.

———. (2004b). Developing the social relational in the social model of disability: A theoretical agenda. In C. Barnes and G. Mercer (Eds.), *Implementing the social model of disability: Theory and research* (pp. 32–47). Leeds: Disability Press.

Thomas, G. M. (2021). Dis-mantling stigma: Parenting disabled children in an age of "neoliberal-ableism." *Sociological Review, 69*(2), 451–467.

Thomas-MacLean, R. (2004). Understanding breast cancer stories via Frank's narrative types. *Social Science & Medicine, 58*(9), 1647–1657.

Thornton Dill, B. (1994). *Across the boundaries of race and class: An exploration of work and family among black female domestic servants.* New York: Garland.

Traustadottir, R. (1991). Mothers who care: Gender, disability, and family life. *Journal of Family Issues, 12*(2), 211–228.

Tronto, J. (1993). *Moral boundaries: A political argument for an ethic of care.* New York: Routledge.

———. (1998). An ethic of care. *Generations, 22*, 15–20.

Tronto, J., & Fisher, B. (1990). Towards a feminist theory of caring. In E. K. Abel and M. K. Nelson (Eds.), *Circles of care: Work and identity in women's lives* (pp. 36–54). Albany: State University of New York Press.

Trottier, G., Srivastava, L., & Walker, C. D. (1999). Etiology of infantile autism: A review of recent advances in genetic and neurobiological research. *Journal of Psychiatry Neuroscience, 24*(2), 103–115.

Tuominen-Eriksson, A. M., Svensson, Y., & Gunnarsson, R. (2013). Children with disabilities are often misdiagnosed initially and children with neuropsychiatric disorders are referred to adequate resources 30 months later than children with other disabilities. *Journal of Autism Developmental Disorder, 43*(3), 579–584.

UPIAS. (1976). *Fundamental principles of disability.* London: Union of the Physically Impaired Against Segregation.

Valentine, K. (2010). A consideration of medicalisation: Choice, engagement and other responsibilities of parents of children with autism spectrum disorder. *Social Science & Medicine, 71*(5), 950–957.

Weiss, J. A. (2003). Self-injurious behaviours in autism: A literature review. *Journal on Developmental Disabilities, 9*(2), 127–144.

Whitehead, L. C. (2006). Quest, chaos and restitution: Living with chronic fatigue syndrome/myalgic encephalomyelitis. *Social Science & Medicine, 62*(9), 2236–2245.

Williams, Gareth. (2000). Knowledgeable narratives. *Anthropology & Medicine, 7*(1), 135–140.

Wing, L. (1981). Asperger's syndrome: A clinical account. *Psychological Medicine, 11*(1), 115–129.

Yergeau, M. (2018). *Authoring autism: On rhetoric and neurological queerness.* Durham, NC: Duke University Press.

Index

Abel, Emily, 14
ableism, 4, 66, 134
advocacy care work, 18, 106, 126
Allen, Katherine, 13
Allies and Obstacles (Carey, Block, and Scotch), 110
alternative communication (AAC) devices, 35
American family. *See* family
Anderson, Laura, 36
anxiety, 29, 57, 59, 79, 84, 87
Applied Behavioral Analysis (ABA) therapy: caregivers and, 93; cost of, 12; critics of, 31; duration of, 30–31, 49; recommendation of, 75, 85; risks associated with, 36
Asperger, Hans, 26–27
Asperger's syndrome, 27, 28, 139
attention deficit hyperactivity disorder (ADHD): behaviour of children with, 95–96; clinical study of, 96; diagnosis of, 29; medicalization of, 18; strengths associated with, 34
autism: among boys and girls, 139; biomedical model of, 24, 25, 26, 29–31, 112, 124, 134; causes of, 29–30; cognitive functions and, 31–32; definitions of, 2; efforts to demedicalize, 120–121; as family issue, 118–119; FDA-approved medications for, 30; history of, 40; institutional practices, 19; medical model of, 4–5, 130; paradigms for understanding, 28–29;

private framework of, 118–119; psychological explanation for, 25; public perception of, 23–24, 47, 52, 53, 56, 58, 67, 101, 112, 121; schizophrenia and, 24, 25; social model of, 19, 31–34, 66, 124; statistics of, 2; symptoms of, 29, 40, 68, 69
autism awareness events, 98, 99–100, 101
autism carework, 3, 11, 14–16, 48–49, 57, 90
autism family social groups, 64
"autism gene," 30
autism interventions: biomedical, 30–31, 36; diet and supplements, 83–85; gender and, 37; medications, 30; neurodiversity-affirming, 35–37; resources for, 35
autism spectrum disorder, 27, 28
autism training, 97, 104–105
autistic children: behaviors of, 41–42, 53–54, 71, 72, 74, 92, 96; bullying experiences, 87, 103; common health issues, 79, 81, 84; evaluation of, 76, 96; everyday activities of, 53; high-cost interventions, 48–49; hypersensitivity of, 55–56; interests and strengths, 60; lack of understanding of, 5, 52–54, 58; leisure activities, 57–58; parents and, 67–68; pediatricians and, 74–76; in public spaces, 55, 56; repetitive behaviors, 72; schooling of, 48, 69, 87–88, 96–97; tantrums of, 59, 71, 83; therapies for, 48, 68, 85;

161

trick-or-treating experience, 54–55;
uncertainty about the future of, 46;
verbal communication of, 52, 72–74
autistic psychopathy, 26–27

Barker, Kristin, 121
Becerra, Walter Suarez, 106
becoming process, 22
Bertilsdotter-Rosqvist, Hanna, 34
Bettelheim, Bruno, 25
biomedical model of disability, 2, 20, 29–31, 112–113
bipolar disorder, 29
Bleuler, Eugen, 24
Block, Pamela, 110
Blum, Linda, 18, 106
Bogida, Eugene, 127
Bourdieu, Pierre, 91
Bury, Michael, 39

California: developmental services, 108; special education, 103
Cancian, Francesca, 15
caregivers: advocacy for autism training, 104–105; agency of, 61, 131; anxieties of, 55, 114–115; "audience member" position of, 114; community outreach, 97–98; demographics, 139–140, 141–143; domestic labor and, 79, 86, 88; feelings of shame, 119; fundraising efforts, 106; gender connotations, 115; grant writing efforts, 106; health literacy of, 84, 93; identity ruptures, 20, 42–44, 57, 58, 65–66; institutional barriers, 104; lack of support, 5–6, 21; as lay diagnosticians, 73, 75; medicalization and, 7, 19, 120, 122; methodological implications of study of, 144; negative attention to, 56; personal endeavors, 97; positionality of, 9; psychological stress, 56–57; as "pushy parents," 113; record keeping, 83; resources, 63, 64; responsibilities of, 12–13; roles and skill sets, 6, 69–70, 81–82, 92–94; self-education, 84; social exclusion of, 9, 43, 44, 58, 119; stories of, 19–22; stress of, 51; study of, 10, 145–146; support networks, 63–65, 91. *See also* expert caregivers

carework: definition of, 14–15, 126; expansion of, 18; fathers' involvement in, 15, 50–51, 88, 144; feminist view of, 125, 128; in formal institutional spheres, 124; gendered distribution of, 16–17, 49–50, 129, 135; intensification of, 1, 17–19, 91, 133, 134; invisibility of, 14, 125, 129, 134; lack of acknowledgment and support, 15, 80; mechanisms of, 126; nurturant framework, 15, 16, 126; outsourcing of, 88; as personal practice, 21; as public practice, 98–99; relationality of, 16; reward for, 15; structural challenges of, 135
Carey, Allison, 110
Centers for Disease Control and Prevention (CDC), 2
Charmaz, Kathy, 39
child behavior: typical *vs.* atypical, 8, 71, 72
chronic illness narratives, 38, 39
cochlear implant technology, 121
community carework: administrative tasks, 100, 101, 123; advocacy in, 104, 106, 122, 123; autism awareness events, 99–100; benefits of, 6–7, 101–102, 106–107, 123; caregivers' attitude to, 107, 118–119; conceptualization of, 21, 99, 106, 107; costs associated with, 101; direct-action measures, 111; engagement practices, 121, 122; event-planning tasks, 101; families of color and, 117; fear to lose support in, 114; gender and, 115; individual carework and, 116; institutional engagement in, 107, 109; labor intensity of, 115; language barriers in, 117; levels of engagement in, 99, 100; limits to, 109, 113–120, 124; medical authority and, 122; mothers and, 100,

102, 123–124; motivation for, 98, 100, 123; politics and, 108, 109–110, 113, 124; as public project, 101, 122, 123; in schools, 102–107; scope of, 98, 102; transformative potentials of, 109–113
community support groups, 63–65
concerted cultivation, 126
Conrad, Peter, 117, 120
coordinated care, 94, 133
cultural capital, 91–92

Davies, Celia, 16, 127
deaf children, 121
demedicalization, 19, 120, 130–131
depression, 29, 57, 84
devaluation framework, 14–15
DeVault, Marjorie, 17
diagnosis of autism: age of receiving, 67, 70; denial of, 52, 53; diagnostic moment, 5, 42; difficulties of, 70, 76; *DSM* guidelines, 25–28, 139; evidence-based practices, 35; history of, 24–27; impact on families, 44–46, 48; medical, 5, 34; mothers and, 66, 76–77; snowball effect of, 47–48, 51, 63; "wait-and-see" approach, 75–76
Diagnostic and Statistical Manual of Mental Disorders (DSM), 25–28
diet, 83, 84–85
disability: definitions of, 32, 33, 38; dominant constructions of, 18–19; idea of "fixing" of, 4; impairment and, 38; sociology of, 38–40; statistics of, 2
disability rights in education, 103
disability studies, 34
Douglas, Patty, 25, 37
Duffy, Mignon, 15
dyslexia, 34

early intensive behavioral therapy (EIBI), 31
Early Start Denver Model, 31
Engels, Friedrich, 14
England, Paula, 14, 15
equine therapy, 48

expert caregivers: access to resources, 12, 91; advocacy for health care reform, 132–133; conceptualization of, 113; as demedicalizing force, 7, 130–131; emergence of, 20, 42, 44; employment of, 133–134; engagement in carework possess, 124; health care bureaucracy and, 69, 76, 80, 91; health literacy skills, 69, 77–81, 90, 92, 127; identity ruptures, 128, 132, 133; knowledge of, 81–82, 130, 131; as lay diagnosticians, 42, 69, 70, 71–76; lay-professional boundaries, 83, 88–91; positionality of, 9; process of becoming, 1–2, 3, 4, 70, 76–77, 80, 90, 126, 131; responsibilities of, 1, 3; as scientific observers, 69; self-confidence of, 61–62, 89–90, 131, 132; social relationships, 7, 128; structural invisibilities of, 131; as teachers, 69, 89; as therapists, 69, 85–87, 89; toolkit of, 77–81, 91, 94, 132
expert carework: all consuming nature of, 128; definition of, 6; distinct quality associated with, 99, 102, 123; dynamics of, 19; emancipatory aspect, 126–128; empowerment of, 128; factors constraining practice of, 21, 109; in institutional spheres, 113; at micro level, 20; outcome of, 132; paradoxes of, 126–131; social context of, 22; systemic inequalities and, 126–127, 129; *vs.* traditional caregiving, 66, 69

families with disabilities: caregiving tasks in, 49–50; decision-making load, 61–62; diversity of, 10; economic disruptions, 47–49, 66; heartwarming events, 59–60; holidays, 53; housing changes, 48, 66; nighttime routine, 59; public perception of, 43; relationship strains, 48, 50–54, 61–62; social interactions, 9, 51–52, 54–55, 58, 63, 65; study of, 10–11; support system for, 93
family: cultural ideals of, 9, 46–47, 129; disruption of narratives of, 44–46;

Index 163

family (*Continued*)
  gendered division of labor in, 88.
  See also traditional nuclear family
feminist ethic of care, 125
fibromyalgia support groups, 121
Finkelstein, Vic, 33
Fox, Renee, 130
Frank, Arthur, 44; *The Wounded
  Storyteller,* 38
Furedi, Frank, 130

gastrointestinal (GI) disturbances, 79, 81
gendered power dynamics, 16–17, 129
Gibson, Margaret, 25, 37
Gluten Free Casein Free (GFCF) diet, 84
"good mothering," 106, 129
Gray, David, 39
Green, Sara, 63

Hays, Sharon, 17
health care: advocacy for reform of, 132–133
health literacy, 69–70, 77–81, 84, 92, 93
Health Resources and Services Administration (HRSA), 2
hypersensitivities, 29

ideology: intensive feeding, 126; spheres of, 127, 128
Individualized Education Plan (IEP), 11, 89, 111, 116, 134
infantile autism, 26
intensive mothering, 17–18, 126
interpretive paradigm for study of clinical narratives, 38
interviews of caregivers: analysis of, 143–144; demographic of participants, 139–140, **141–143**; emotional sharing, 138–139; schedule, 138, 144; settings, 137–138; topics, 138, 139; types of questions, 140
invisible disabilities, 22, 53, 63, 75

K-12 schools: autism training, 104–105; autistic children in, 35–36, 69, 96–97;
bullying in, 87, 103; community carework and, 102–107; safety plan, 103; special education plans, 103–104, 111
Kanner, Leo, 24, 25, 26
Kibria, Nazli, 106
Kleinman, Arthur, 38

Landsman, Gail, 60
Lareau, Annette, 92
lay diagnosticians, 70, 71, 73, 75, 77, 79
lay epidemiology, 81
Litt, Jacquelyn, 18, 106
Lovaas, Ole Ivar, 30, 31, 37

Marx, Karl, 14
Mauldin, Laura, 121
McGill, Owen, 36
Medical Academy of Pediatric Special Needs program (MAPS), 89
medicalese, 82–83, 127
medicalization: of atypical children, 18; of autism, 117, 118; caregivers as agents of, 120; "double-edged sword" of, 21, 109, 121, 129; duality of, 131; levels of, 117–118; shortcomings of, 120–124
Miller, Andrea, 127
Mishler, Elliott, 38
Modified Checklist for Autism in Toddlers-Revised (M-CHAT-R), 71
mothers: access to resources, 11, 116; blame of, 18–19; as caregivers, 7–8, 13, 16–17, 18, 50, 53–54, 89; decision-making, 61–62; domestic labor, 79; employment of, 10, 133–134; experiences in public spaces, 56; gendered stereotypes, 13–14, 17, 127, 128–129; health literacy, 77, 78–79, 80–81; lack of support, 8; as lay diagnosticians, 73–74, 75, 79; letter-writing campaigns, 110; lifestyle, 58; political organizing work, 109; professional and educational background, 11, 109, 111,

116; psychological distress, 86, 128; sacrifices in careers and personal life, 128; social disadvantage, 12, 16–17, 66; stories of, 69; studies of, 60–61, 106; traditional expectations from, 42–43; transformation to stay-at-home, 57, 58

narrative wreckage, 44
Nelson, Margaret, 14
neurodivergence, 18–19, 70, 121
neurodivergent-affirming therapies, 35
neurodiversity framework, 20, 34–37
neurotypical brains, 31, 32

obsessive compulsive disorder, 29
occupational therapy (OT), 11, 48, 49, 75, 85, 86, 93
Oliker, Stacey, 15
Oliver, Michael, 32, 33

parental disability activism, 110
Pervasive Developmental Disorders (PDD), 26
physical therapy (PT), 11, 48, 49, 85, 86, 93
popular epidemiology, 81
private therapies, 12, 76
prosocial practices, 109
"pushy parents," 113–114, 115, 117

"refrigerator mother," 25
Riessman, Catherine, 121
reproductive labor, 14
Robinson, Anna, 36

Scotch, Richard, 110
sensory seeking behaviors, 73
Shakespeare, Tom, 38
Shook, Natalie, 119
Singer, Judy, 34
Singh, Jennifer, 18; *Multiple Autisms*, 30
Skinner, B. F., 30

sleep disturbances, 29, 81, 83–84
Smith, Dorothy, 8, 42
social and communication disorder (SCD), 27
social capital, 91
social model of disability: autism and, 31–34; conceptualization of, 2, 20, 28, 32–33; debate over, 33, 38; social-relational aspect in, 33–34; *vs.* "wounded storyteller" paradigm, 39
special education systems, 103–104, 106
speech therapy: for autistic children, 48, 68, 69, 73, 74, 93, 127; frequency of, 86; insurance coverage of, 85; play-based, 12, 80
Standard North American Family (SNAF), 8–9, 42–43, 45
Stenning, Anna, 34
street science, 81
supplements, 83–84, 85
support networks, 63–65
symbolic resources, 9, 43, 63, 64, 65

Terrizzi, John, 119
Thomas, Carol, 33
traditional nuclear family, 8, 9, 42–43, 45–46, 62, 116, 129
Tronto, Joan, 126

Union of the Physically Impaired Against Segregation (UPIAS), 32

Valentine, Kylie, 90
Vigilante Mothers, 126
vitamins, 83–84

Walker, Alexis, 13
Watson, Nicholas, 38
Wing, Lorna, 27
"wounded storyteller" paradigm, 39

Zola, Irving, 39

Index   165

About the Author

CARA A. CHIARALUCE is Teaching Professor of Sociology at Santa Clara University. She conducts research at the intersections of carework, family, disability, and health.